ayurveda
MADE EASY

50 Exercises *for* Finding
Health, Mindfulness,
and Balance

Heidi E. Spear

Adams Media
New York   London   Toronto   Sydney   New Delhi

A adamsmedia

Adams Media
An Imprint of Simon & Schuster, Inc.
57 Littlefield Street
Avon, Massachusetts 02322

First Adams Media hardcover edition
AUGUST 2017

Library of Congress Cataloging-in-Publication Data
Spear, Heidi E., author.
Ayurveda made easy / Heidi E. Spear.
Avon, Massachusetts: Adams Media, 2017.
Includes index.
LCCN 2017017304 (print) | LCCN 2017022330 (ebook) | ISBN 9781507204399 (hc) | ISBN 9781507204405 (ebook)
LCSH: Medicine, Ayurvedic. | Holistic medicine. | BISAC: HEALTH & FITNESS / Alternative Therapies. | HEALTH & FITNESS / Healthy Living. | HEALTH & FITNESS / General.
LCC R605 (ebook) | LCC R605 .S72 2017 (print) | DDC 615.5/38--dc23
LC record available at https://lccn.loc.gov/2017017304

ISBN 978-1-5072-0439-9
ISBN 978-1-5072-0440-5 (ebook)

For information about special discounts for bulk purchases, please contact Simon & Schuster Special Sales at 1-866-506-1949 or business@simonandschuster.com.

The Simon & Schuster Speakers Bureau can bring authors to your live event. For more information or to book an event contact the Simon & Schuster Speakers Bureau at 1-866-248-3049 or visit our website at www.simonspeakers.com.

Interior design by Colleen Cunningham
Yoga pose images by Eric Andrews

Manufactured in the United States of America

10 9 8 7 6 5 4 3 2

Sudha Carolyn Lundeen, RN, Ayurvedic health and lifestyle coach, and 200- and 500-hour yoga teacher trainer at Kripalu Center in Massachusetts, designed the breathwork section and yoga sequence for vata types. Contact her at www.sudhalundeen.com to order her *Taming the Winds of Vata* CD that guides you through another yoga sequence for balancing vata dosha.

The yoga and pranayama sequences are designed for pitta types by Janna Delgado, a yoga and Ayurvedic specialist at Kripalu Center for Yoga & Health.

Contains material adapted from the following titles published by Adams Media, an Imprint of Simon & Schuster, Inc.: *The Everything® Guide to Ayurveda* by Heidi E. Spear, copyright © 2012, ISBN 978-1-4405-2996-2 and *Adaptogens* by Agatha Noveille, copyright © 2016, ISBN 978-1-4405-9639-1.

Contents

Introduction

Would you like to flow through life with greater ease, contentment, mental clarity, and physical health? Would you like to feel a sense of empowerment and understanding when it comes to your overall well-being? Are you interested in preventing disease before it develops, knocks you down, or becomes life-threatening? If so, Ayurveda is for you. Ayurveda addresses the vitality of your entire being—body, mind, and life-force energy—for a life of balance, sustainable health, and longevity.

Ayurveda, often translated as "the science of life," can also be considered "universal knowledge." More simply put, it is an "owner's manual" that teaches you how to keep yourself running well day in and day out. Just as other creatures are wired into natural rhythms in nature such as hibernation or migration patterns, the human being, or *Homo sapiens*, is wired with particular rhythms as well. The more you align with your natural rhythms, the more balanced and harmonious you are, and the more harmonious the world becomes. These premises sit strongly in the system of Ayurvedic medicine and guide every aspect of existence.

Ayurveda teaches us the tools of living well in easy, practical ways; how to correct imbalances through simple changes to daily routines, food choices, exercise; and the use of natural herbal formulas or treatment protocols. Ayurveda is not only a science but a complete medical system based on sound principles of science, and as a system of medicine spanning thousands of years, it not only carries the knowledge base forward rooted in science, but it also can verify its effectiveness through its repeated applications and verifiable results that have been tried and true for all these many years.

Ayurveda Made Easy is a great place to start your journey. It will help you find your own balance through the lens and guidance of Ayurveda.

PART I

The Science of Life

1

What Is Ayurveda?

A Complete Medical System

Ayurveda is a holistic, natural system of health, originating in India more than 5,000 years ago. Perhaps the oldest extant medical system in the world, Ayurveda's teachings are timeless. Now, when looking for natural, holistic, and safe ways to create health for themselves and their families, people all over the world are looking to Ayurveda for its vast knowledge base, effective treatments, and practical ideas. Ayurveda offers remedies for illness, and is designed as a preventive medicine that supports consistent health and longevity.

Ayurveda is a complete medical system. It treats the whole person as an integrated being: body, mind, and spirit. Ayurveda is a comprehensive medical system that includes: surgery, psychotherapy, pediatrics, gynecology, obstetrics, ophthalmology, geriatrics, ear/nose/throat, and general medicine. All of these branches are subsumed in the holistic practice of Ayurveda, which takes into consideration all aspects of your life, and employs a variety of healing modalities to support your health and help you thrive day by day, year by year.

Ayurveda's diet and lifestyle approaches are simple and basic, and "one step at a time" is a great way to approach it if it feels like too much at once. As a science, Ayurveda actually makes sense, and you'll be able to notice when you're sliding out of balance. Then, you can turn to Ayurvedic guidance to keep yourself healthy year-round. You also can have fun with it—customizing recipes, and enjoying its natural and life-affirming recommendations. It's a whole new way to view health—in a positive way that supports the lifestyle your body, mind, and spirit desire.

Nonspecialized Treatment

Ayurveda doesn't specialize, which means it doesn't focus on healing just one organ or one symptom at a time. As a holistic practice, Ayurveda creates overall health, recognizing that body, mind, and spirit are interrelated. So, its goal is twofold:

1. To alleviate the discomfort of something like a headache, stomachache, or cold, and
2. To bring you into balance to prevent those symptoms from recurring and worsening.

When you start to get sick, if you choose not to make changes in your diet and lifestyle and instead only take allopathic drugs for the symptoms, it's likely that your symptoms will worsen and/or recur. In Ayurveda, the idea is to create harmony in your mind, body, and spirit so your body can support its own healing and become well enough to discourage recurring symptoms and the development of disease.

Your body wants to be well, and it's designed to function in harmony with the natural world. To create health, your body must be able to perform its vital functions, which include the absorption of vitamins and minerals, and the elimination of toxins. Rather than just suggesting a quick fix, Ayurveda gives you the tools to create a state of harmony in your body and mind so that your body can perform its required functions to keep you healthy.

Each Moment, Each Choice Counts

Ayurveda is a way of living. It's about being healthy from moment to moment. As you wake up in the morning, as you eat your meals, as you schedule in time for exercise and play, Ayurveda teaches you to consider what nourishes your mind, body, and spirit.

What you eat, what you watch on Netflix, how much time you spend exchanging the energy of love with others—everything you do, say, think, and feel has an impact on your body, mind, and energy system.

Each moment you make a choice. You can choose to do something that helps create balance in you or that may bring you out of balance. Ayurveda gives you knowledge about yourself and your relationship to the external world so that you can make informed choices each moment, each meal, each day, and each season.

Your health will improve as you make one choice at a time—what to eat, what to think, what to wear, when to exercise, whom to hang out with, how to manage your reactions. You have choices. If it seems as though you don't have time or energy to make new choices, think about this: You can make one small change at a time. And notice how it makes you feel. Then, decide if you'd like to incorporate another change. Go at your own pace. Keep remembering that you are the one who decides how to take care of yourself. It's up to you.

A Brief History of Ayurveda

Ayurveda is Sanskrit for "the science of life." *Ayur* means "life," and *veda* means "to know," or "knowledge." So, Ayurveda is the knowledge of what it is to be living, of how to live healthily and in harmony with this planet and all that is. More than 5,000 years ago, rishis, or "seers of truth," passed down the knowledge of Ayurveda only to their students as an oral tradition. Now, Ayurveda has become a part of the consciousness of the mainstream Western lifestyle.

The Beginnings of Ayurveda

In a way very different from many modern Western medical discoveries, Ayurveda didn't originate in laboratories or research centers. While in meditative states, rishis in India began to understand the nature of life, health, and longevity that has come to be what we call Ayurveda.

More than 2,000 years ago, much of Ayurveda's wisdom was transcribed into Sanskrit. Many of those texts are still around today. Today, Ayurvedic specialists learn from the wisdom of these texts and from the wisdom of practitioners who combine that knowledge with their proven experience in Ayurveda and allopathic, or traditional Western, medicine.

You Have the Same Elements As the Eternal Cosmos

One of the philosophers of this age, Kapila, is credited with the philosophy of creation known as Samkhya from the roots *sat*, meaning "truth," and *kyah*, meaning "to know." This "knowledge of truth" is the foundation of Ayurveda. According to Samkhya philosophy, before physical matter existed there were two eternal forces:

1. Consciousness that is pure awareness, called *Purusha*. Purusha is considered the male energy of the universe. It is the universal intelligence and consciousness that just is.

2. A force of creativity/action called *Prakruti*. Prakruti is considered the female energy of the universe, which is awareness plus choice and the desire for creation. It is from the energy of Prakruti that the universe, and each human being, has come into existence.

Samkhya explains that each human being is a microcosm of the macrocosm (the universe). Each person's physical makeup is a combination of the five elements of the universe. Everyone is individual in her constitutional makeup, and is always in relationship with the energy and elements outside of herself. So, Ayurveda looks at health in terms of the individual's constitution and how to keep that in balance with the changing external elements.

Your Relationship to the Cosmos

Here is the story of creation according to the rishis who realized Samkhya philosophy: Before the creation of life on earth, there existed two eternal cosmic forces: Purusha (pure awareness) and Prakruti (creative energy). Everything that is created comes from Prakruti, and Purusha is the eternal witness, with no participation in creation.

Prakruti is energy that contains the three gunas, or attributes:

1. Sattva (creative potential)
2. Tamas (inertia or destructive potential)
3. Rajas (movement/kinetic force), in balance

AYURVEDA WORKS WITH RELIGIONS

Ayurveda's nontheistic creation story is compatible with theistic beliefs. If you believe in a God or creator, it's also possible to incorporate the realization that you are made of the same elements that you experience outside. Samkhya philosophy explains that your physical and energetic bodies are comprised of the same elements as the natural world.

One by One, the Elements Formed

From Prakruti, the force of creation, the soundless vibration "aum" began to stir. "Aum" is said to be the first energetic vibration, from which all else is born. All matter is energy at its basic unit, and "aum" is the first vibration of energy.

The vibration "aum" had to be vibrating somewhere. It was vibrating in space; that's how the rishis realized the element ether. When the element of ether began to move, it created air, the element of movement. As air began to move, it created friction, which creates heat, the element of fire. Fire has the property of transformation. Because of fire's transforming property it caused elements of ether to liquefy into water, and coalesce into matter, earth. From the earth, all living matter is created, grows, and returns. This includes all the food that is nourishing to you, the water you drink, and vitamins and minerals you get from the air you breathe and the sunshine you soak up. You are of the elements, and you thrive and grow based on your relationship to them. Living in harmony with the elements keeps you healthy, youthful, and balanced. Ayurveda contains simple, natural, and fun ways to achieve this balance.

Ayurveda for the English-Speaking World

Once only available to those indigenous to India, Ayurveda now is available to the English-speaking world through various textbooks, guides, websites, and cookbooks. In addition, there are schools of Ayurveda, where students learn through study and practice about the ancient art of Ayurveda and Ayurvedic consulting.

The National Institutes of Health includes Ayurveda among the complementary health systems it researches. The site for the National Center for Complementary and Integrative Health (NCCIH) is: https://nccih.nih.gov.

WHAT IS AYURVIDYA?

Authentic understanding of Ayurveda is said to come from the Ayurvidya. *Ayur* means "life," and *vidya* means "living wisdom." Ayurvidya is personified as the goddess embodying and transmitting the universal wisdom that is Ayurveda. When you practice Ayurveda, you can connect to her healing energy and acknowledge it in the herbs, spices, oils, and foods you prepare.

Your Constitution, the Doshas

Ayurveda assesses your state of being and the state of the natural world in terms of three basic principles, or *doshas*. The doshas are vata, pitta, and kapha:

- Vata is a combination of the elements of ether and air
- Pitta is a combination of fire and water
- Kapha is both water and earth elements

According to Ayurveda, your personal type, your constitution, is described by how these doshas were set in you when you were conceived.

All the doshas and elements are a part of you. For most people, one or two of the doshas are most prominent at conception, and that determines their constitution. Some people are tridoshic, which means their constitution is vata-pitta-kapha. Most people are what is called "dual doshic," with two doshas sharing a higher percentage proportionally. So, the other configurations of constitutional types can be vata-pitta, vata-kapha, or pitta-kapha. To nuance a bit further, a person can carry a stronger proportion of one of these so there are also those last three combinations reversed to appear as pitta-vata, kapha-vata, or kapha-pitta.

DOSHA, DEFINED TWO WAYS

The word *dosha* has two meanings. Dosha shows up in the ancient texts as the way of naming the three principles (vata, pitta, kapha). Vata, pitta, and kapha, when in balance, are the actual tissues and components of your body (dhatus). When vata, pitta, or kapha are imbalanced, dosha can also mean "impure," i.e., "vata is dosha."

Your original constitution is called your prakruti. Your Ayurvedic practitioner (see Part 3) can figure out your prakruti by pulse diagnosis, and you can learn to tell which doshas are active in you once you learn which qualities are associated with each element and how to notice them in yourself. Month to month, and even hour by hour, you may notice changes in how you feel the doshas are at work inside of you.

When you are out of balance, the relationship of vata-pitta-kapha in you is called your *vikruti*. For health, you want to be in balance, which means that the relationship of vata, pitta, kapha is balanced in you in the same way it was when you were born. Various lifestyle and dietary habits can bring you out of balance, and you will learn to be able to notice in you when that is happening and how to steer yourself back toward balance.

The Qualities in Nature

Each dosha is described as a combination of two elements, and each element is described according to its qualities. Ayurveda lists twenty observable qualities. These qualities are expressed as ten sets of opposites: hot/cold, oily/dry, rough/smooth (slimy), heavy/light, soft/hard, static/mobile, cloudy/clear, gross/subtle, slow/sharp, liquid/solid (dense). The following table shows how Ayurveda describes each dosha and its qualities.

Dosha	Associated Qualities
Vata	dry, light, cold, rough, subtle, mobile, clear
Pitta	hot, sharp, light, liquid, mobile, oily
Kapha	heavy, slow, cold, oily, liquid, smooth, dense, soft, static, gross

For example, "solid" is typically associated with kapha because kapha has the element of earth, which is a solid, grounding force. When you feel securely solid in your life, that is a quality of kapha in you *(see image on page 1 of the insert)*.

As you learn more about Ayurveda and start observing qualities in yourself and in nature, you may wonder which qualities go with which dosha, and that's understandable. While you are beginning to practice Ayurveda, it will help to keep these tables handy for reference. You can use both your reasoning skills and these tables to help remember which qualities are associated with which elements and doshas. And, as you do, it will become second nature for you to notice qualities in yourself, and associate it to a particular element.

Why is it important to begin to associate qualities with the elements and doshas? It's foundational to the practice of Ayurveda to see yourself and the world around you in terms of the elements because the way to create health according to Ayurveda is to support the balance of the elements in you. Your constitution, set at birth, is a particular balance of the elements in you that reflects your own unique nature. Each individual will have slightly different elemental proportions. Maintaining your unique nature and balance of these elements is the state of health for you, and the state in which you will be well and live a long, healthy life. It is common to talk about the constitutional types through the language of the doshas, but it is important to see it more properly through the concept of the elements. For the purposes of simplicity you can begin to identify constitutional types through this paradigm: vata as ether and air, pitta as fire and water, and kapha as water and earth.

How to Recognize the Qualities in You

The following checklists are examples of how you can begin to notice how vata, pitta, and kapha are showing up in you. These checklists are to help you start to get the idea of how to observe yourself in terms of the qualities. These brief checklists are not to be used for diagnosis. They are here to give you a sense of what kinds of behaviors and patterns you'll be observing in yourself, as you begin to understand your state of health according to the doshas.

Vata

Vata is made up of air and space. This combination of elements is the force behind many vital functions in the body, including the functioning of the heart and circulatory system. Vata also helps fan the fire of digestion and aids in elimination. Its energy is necessary for the workings of the mind and intellect. Through its vital role in the functions of the heart, mind, gut, and intellect, vata helps you experience your deepest wisdom and brightest knowing.

Vata is located in and as the space in the open cavities of the body, such as the spaces in between bones and joints—particularly in the lower back, pelvic area, and hips. Its primary site is the colon.

VATA'S SUBTLE ENERGY: PRANA

Prana is vital life-force energy. It's likened to the concept of *chi* in Chinese medicine and *qi* in Japanese culture. Prana is an essential factor in your well-being, and yoga and Ayurveda help you understand, move, and work with prana. The natural and whole foods you eat contain prana, the sun contains prana, the exercise and rest you take helps prana flow, and breathwork and yoga help you consciously move life-force energy through your mind and body.

The physical characteristics of vata are a thin, light frame; dry skin and hair; cold hands and feet; and a sensitive digestive system. Those with more vata are likely to sleep lightly. When vata is out of balance, a variety of uncomfortable symptoms can occur, from dry mouth to constipation. And the longer vata is left unchecked, the more wear and tear your body will experience from the inside out. When you keep vata in balance, there are so many wonderful mental and physical processes it supports, from expansive and creative thinking to proper biological functions.

OBSERVING VATA
○ Do you talk quickly and often?
○ Do you often feel anxious?
○ Are you constipated?
○ Are you more comfortable seeing the big picture rather than the small details?
○ Do you easily feel connected to spiritual and energetic existence?

These questions help you determine if vata is working strongly in you. Talking quickly and often and feeling anxious have the "mobile" or "movement" quality of vata. If you're constipated, that points to the dry quality of vata. And if you tend to be more comfortable seeing the larger picture in life, instead of focusing on small details, that shows the spacious/ether quality of vata. If you easily and comfortably tap into the spiritual and creative worlds, that connection is an expression of the subtle, ethereal quality of vata.

Pitta

Being able to effectively and efficiently complete tasks shows the "sharp" quality of the pitta mind and the fiery quality of pitta in action. If you are quick to anger and become critical, that points to the fiery and mobile qualities of pitta. If you are usually hot, even when others around you are not, that shows the hot qualities of pitta. And if you are fanatical in your relationship to spirit or adamant about your stance against the possibility of spirit, that also points to the fiery pitta energy. Remember, pitta is the dosha associated with fire.

Two of the qualities of pitta—fire and fluidity—help you come up with great ideas, accomplish goals, and push projects to completion. The sharpness of the pitta mind loves to achieve, and the fiery momentum helps burn through obstacles to that end.

The physical attributes of pitta can be: reddish hair or baldness; moderate body; freckles; sharp eyes that are brown, hazel, or green. Pittas usually are of moderate build. But remember you don't need to have all these qualities to have a good deal of pitta in your constitution. These are simple ways of viewing the likelihood of pitta being present.

It's very important for a pitta person who is on the move and on a mission (whether in business or with family) to keep her pitta balanced so she doesn't start to get too pushy, angry, annoyed, and judgmental. While it is exciting and creates a great sense of accomplishment to keep up the momentum and fuel the fire, it's important to balance that fire so others will enjoy working with you and supporting you as you reach your goals. You won't cool off too much if you balance your fire: You'll still shine, shine, shine, and you'll do it with more finesse and joy if you don't get yourself overheated.

PITTA'S SUBTLE ENERGY: TEJAS

The subtle force of pitta is tejas. Tejas is responsible for inner glow, clarity, courage, intelligence, and understanding at the cellular level. It's important to keep tejas in balance, and the same methods for balancing pitta will work with tejas. To calm overstimulated tejas, as you would do with pitta, be mindful of your diet, your exercise, and the use of stimulants. When your fire is too hot, you want to cool it down to protect your immune system, your tissues, your organs, and your mind from burnout.

OBSERVING PITTA

◯ Are you able to effectively and efficiently complete tasks?
◯ Are you quick to anger?
◯ Are you highly critical of yourself and others?
◯ Are you usually hot, even when others are neutral or cold?
◯ Are you fanatical in your spiritual, religious, or nonreligious stance?

If you answered "yes" to those questions, you are noticing the signs of pitta in you. Just from this checklist, you aren't making a diagnosis or judgment about whether it's balanced in you or overactive. This checklist is introducing you to some of the ways to notice pitta.

Kapha

Kapha is of the elements earth and water. Kapha's qualities are stable, oily, heavy, dense, smooth, and cool. A kapha type will remind you of Mother Earth: She emanates a nurturing, tolerant energy, with a calming sense of stability.

Physically, kapha types tend to have nice curves and some excess body weight. Their bodies are heavy and strong. Kapha's skin appears soft, smooth, oily, clear, and pale. Their eyes are sensual, black or blue, clear, big, and bright. Hair is blond or jet-black, wavy, shiny, and abundant.

KAPHA'S SUBTLE ENERGY: OJAS

Just as vata and pitta have their subtle energies (prana and tejas, respectively), kapha has a subtle energy: ojas. Ojas is the essence that remains after your digestion and assimilation of food, thoughts, and impressions. If you are able to digest well, then ojas will be sustained in you. It will keep the vital organs and tissues of your body healthy. Ojas provides endurance for both the body and the mind. It is said that among its many sustaining attributes, ojas lubricates the nerves of the nervous system, so nervous breakdowns, for example, signal low ojas.

When trying to determine if you or a loved one has the characteristics of a kapha body, see if any of these descriptions apply: thick muscles, strong bones, large body frame, thick eyelashes, cold skin, large eyes. You might also be prone to gaining weight and to getting congested in the head and chest.

If you say "That's me!" when you read most of these attributes, you are noticing kapha qualities. This isn't enough to determine, yet, if kapha is the only dosha dominant in your constitution. You may have a significant amount of the attributes of another dosha too. Everyone has some of all three doshas at work in the body. So, a more comprehensive Ayurvedic questionnaire, and a meeting with an Ayurvedic specialist, will help you determine how predominant kapha is in your personal constitution.

Kaphas are slow to learn, but once they learn something they will remember it. They are peaceful by nature and very forgiving. Kaphas develop attachments to people and things, which is why they tend to store and save items more than other people will. They can be prone to envy and greed, if kapha is out of balance.

OBSERVING KAPHA
○ Do you gain weight easily and have difficulty losing it?
○ Most of the year, is it hard for you to get moving?
○ Are you prone to depression?
○ Is your sleep heavy and long-lasting?
○ Are you loyal to your friends and loved ones?

This checklist helps you acclimate to noticing the qualities of kapha. Kapha is a grounded, gross (as opposed to subtle) dosha. Being of earth it is hard, steady, and solid. Because of this, it's a stabilizing and nurturing force of life. Ways you may notice it in you could be that you have a larger frame and gain weight easily.

You may have trouble initiating movement or projects because "mobility" is a quality associated with vata and pitta, not kapha. If you're prone to depression it could be a sign of the dense and dull qualities of kapha. If your sleep is heavy and long, that shows deep and slow or lethargic qualities. And your loyalty to friends shows that solid, soft side of kapha.

Recognizing Dosha Imbalance

Vata
There are very clear signs of vata imbalance that you can look out for.

Physical Symptoms of Excess Vata
Vata moves throughout the body, and affects the bones and the colon in particular. Because vata's elements are air and space, when you want to remember the signs of vata imbalance, think of the qualities that go with air and space, such as: cool, dry, light, and mobile.

EARLY PHYSICAL SIGNS OF VATA IMBALANCE
- Dry mouth and dry skin
- Constipation
- Short and shallow breathing
- Cold hands and feet
- Inability to sit still and focus
- Excess gas: burping, hiccoughs, etc.
- Insomnia

When you notice these early signs, you can take action by making sure your diet is vata pacifying, by eating at regular times, and by giving yourself an oil massage at least once per day with sesame oil or specially prepared herbalized oil for vata. If you're experiencing constipation, your specialist might recommend you take the herb triphala, as well.

Emotional and Mental Signs of Vata Imbalance

When vata is in excess, it affects your mental clarity and your emotional balance. There are very easy ways to tell if vata is influencing your state of mind.

MENTAL SIGNS OF VATA IMBALANCE
- Anxiety
- Fear
- Whirling, crowded, and continual stream of thoughts
- Disturbed sleep

When you experience these symptoms, even though they are *mental* symptoms, you can ameliorate them with *physical* practices. So, for example, drinking hot water with lemon, making sure you're eating enough at meals, having some warm milk before bed, practicing vata-pacifying *pranayama* (breath control), and other such actions will help with your mental state.

When vata imbalance continues in the body, it can lead to certain types of arthritis, more serious digestive disorders, chronic lower back pain, and emotional imbalances. So, if you catch the signs of vata imbalance early (for example, when you're experiencing anxiety or constipation), you can use Ayurveda as preventive care.

Practice Noticing Vata

Becoming aware of how vata is showing up in you can take a little bit of practice. You can start to notice how you are doing by taking time throughout the day to pause and observe.

TAKE A MOMENT TO STOP

Here's a simple meditation for you to try. Take time during the day to stop what you're doing, and just take a few moments to notice how you are. Do this daily to check in with yourself *(see images for proper meditation posture on page 2 of the insert)*.

DAILY FIVE-MINUTE CHECK-IN

1. Log off of the computer. And turn off your cell phone.
2. Sit down, and sit up straight. Place your feet firmly on the floor. Roll your shoulders up, back, and down. Close your eyes.
3. Notice your breath. Is it shallow, short, long, deep? Watch the breath, without changing it.
4. After you notice your breath, focus lightly on it.
5. Notice the mind's activity for several breaths. As thoughts come up, allow them to float by. Return your focus lightly to the breath, so you don't get caught up in your mind's activity.
6. After watching the thoughts for several breaths, take a nice deep inhalation and let it out on a longer exhalation.
7. Return to normal breathing, and reflect on how your thoughts were: nervous, anxious, spinning, foggy, clear, optimistic?

If after this exercise you notice that you are experiencing a lot of anxiety, fear, and worry, this is something to pay attention to. Everyone's mind will have thoughts during that type of meditation. It's natural for the mind to keep thinking. And you can pay attention to it and see if it's predominantly worried, foggy, or generally clear. If you notice you're experiencing anxiety and worry, try a vata-pacifying diet, plan some soothing activities, and hang out with supportive friends or family. And, most of all, do not judge yourself for having excess vata. With many to-dos and a culture that encourages fast-paced living and fast-paced eating, it's no wonder you may have excess vata.

Prevent Vata Imbalance

If you can keep vata pacified without waiting to see signs of imbalance, that is best. If you know you have a lot of vata in your constitution, then it won't be a surprise to you that during certain times of day, certain times of year, and later in life, you will need to be especially conscious of vata dosha.

Since vata time of day is 2–6 p.m. (and 2–6 a.m.), do your best to avoid activities that can make you stirred up or anxious during those hours. Try breathwork and yoga for vata at that time of day. Or soak in a hot bath, give yourself a soothing massage, or take a nap. You don't have to spend the whole four hours from 2–6 p.m. doing very soothing things, but try to do something calming for vata during those hours each day. Be mindful during vata time of day, and take breaks when you can.

ASHWAGANDHA FOR VATA BALANCE
Talk to your Ayurvedic specialist about herbs for vata time of year if you are prone to vata imbalance. She may recommend you take ashwagandha, which can address some vata disorders including joint discomfort and anxiety. Talk to your specialist about dosage and if it would be right for you.

Because the fall and winter are vata times of year and your later years of life are vata years, these are times in your life to be particularly aware of how you are affected. Do what you can to stay warm: drink plenty of warm liquids, give yourself warm oil massages at least once per day, eat warm foods, and calm your mind. The darkness of the wintertime can aid meditation and introspection, so use that to your advantage. Calming the mind and warming the body is especially important during vata season and vata time of life. Because you know this, you can start taking care of vata before you notice particular imbalances.

Enjoy the Benefits of Vata

It's very important to keep an eye on yourself to see if vata is out of balance. It's also important to be grateful for the wonderful aspects of vata—all of the bodily functions it assists (including the workings of the heart and circulatory system), and how it helps the mind and your connection to higher levels of consciousness. So take time, while being careful to balance vata, to also appreciate it for all it offers with its movement, expansiveness, and airy qualities.

Pitta

When you wonder about what excess pitta could look like for the mind and body, think about the effects of heat. Imagine what effects flowing heat could have on the insides of your body (since pitta is hot and fluid).

How to Recognize Pitta Imbalance

A person who is hotheaded is known to be easily angered, and can fly off the handle without much warning. To others, a hotheaded person's reactions can seem unfounded, unwarranted, and too much to handle. Too much pitta also affects the mind, causing it to experience jealousy and control issues, which can be detrimental to relationships in work and in the home. When pitta is in excess, you can become domineering and hard to please.

If your pitta is out of control, all that fire is a lot for your body and mind to experience. If you are predominantly pitta and your pitta is in excess, you may not realize that it's not healthy to be constantly hot, pushing, and exerting yourself. It does take a toll, over the long haul, on your health.

Also, if you are hard to please and controlling, it affects your ability to experience a deep sense of love, trust, and joy when in a relationship (work or otherwise) with others. By balancing your pitta, you could open up to a more collaborative and harmonious existence in your work and home life . . . and still be outstandingly productive.

Physical Symptoms of Pitta Imbalance

A good way to remember what effects pitta has on the physical body is to think of it as though there were molten lava in the body. Imagine how molten lava spurts and spreads from a volcano. So, when pitta is aggravated, it can lead to such things as acne, rash, ulcers, heartburn, loose stools, and excess urine. And due to pitta's spreading nature, one may find it spilling into other parts of the body, as well.

A Quiz about Your Pitta

It may be hard for you to recognize if your pitta is in excess, especially if you are used to living that way. Take a moment to answer these questions:

- Do you compare yourself to others, feeling competitive in nature?
- Are you often irritated with your family members or close friends?
- Do you look at what your colleagues or coworkers are doing and think of ways they could be doing their job better?
- Does it bother you if the books on your shelf aren't organized in exactly the way you think is best?
- Are you often sure that your way is the right way?

Be honest with yourself when you answer these questions. If you answer yes to many of them, you may want to really make sure that your pitta is in check. Pitta in excess is one reason that a pitta's life span tends to be moderately long, rather than very long. They burn their energy so quickly that what they have will last fewer years. And you could be making the people around you more uncomfortable than you want to, while also adding unnecessary stress to your own life. You are full of potential and brightness, so it can be a struggle to not overdo it.

Enjoy Pitta in Balance

When pitta is in balance, you are a very bright light. You're sleeping well, your digestion is working well, and your mind is sharp and active. You are grounded and secure, and able to accomplish things while also taking time off to relax, play, and be full of compassion.

Kapha

There are physical and emotional signs of kapha imbalance. It's important to balance kapha and catch these signs early because too much kapha engenders a kind of lethargy that can be hard to move through, making it more difficult to get back in balance. Fortunately, as with all doshas, you know what to do: Start doing activities, thinking thoughts, and eating foods that have the opposite qualities that kapha has.

Kapha's Physical Symptoms of Imbalance

When kapha is in excess, you will feel lethargic. You will need naps, you will have a difficult time getting out of bed in the morning, and you will gain weight. You may start to have mucus drainage, coughs, and sinus headaches. A general sense of inertia and inability to motivate yourself to physically move will increase as the kapha tips more and more off balance.

See if these apply to you:

PHYSICAL SIGNS OF YOUR KAPHA IN EXCESS
- You drink at least two cups of coffee during the day, and there is no effect.
- You go to sleep early, you sleep in, and still you're feeling low-energy all day.
- You're craving sweets, eating sweets, and gaining weight.
- Your body is discharging mucus.

GLUTEN AND THE DOSHAS

Gluten intolerance can produce very similar effects to kapha being out of balance, or even other doshas being out of balance. So it's very important to find out what you are allergic to, either by consulting your doctors or by taking things out of your diet and seeing if your symptoms improve. For some people, it's best to avoid gluten.

These could be signs of a kapha imbalance. If you notice these signs, start changing your food choices and activities to balance kapha. The fastest and simplest thing you can do is to modify what you eat: That has an immediate impact on the body. Sometimes you just will be tired and lethargic because you've been burning yourself out. If you aren't sure, give yourself a few days of rest, being sure to hydrate well. If the symptoms persist, this could include both a kapha imbalance and also other issues that need to be addressed. So talk to your doctors and healers if you're noticing lethargy and weight gain.

Kapha's Mental and Emotional Signs of Imbalance

Kapha is by nature loving, caring, grounding, and forgiving, and when kapha is in excess it can turn into jealousy and feelings of needing to cling on to something and someone. If you're starting to feel jealous and clingy, this could be your sign that your kapha is out of balance.

Effects of Long-Term Kapha Imbalance

Every doshic imbalance has particular long-term effects. When kapha is out of balance, it creates the logical kinds of difficulties on the body that you would imagine from its qualities of stable, oily, heavy, dense, smooth, and cool:

- Obesity: If you sit often because of work, if you munch throughout the day on food, watch a lot of TV when you're not working, and sleep a lot, you could very likely be increasing your kapha. You will notice the effects in weight gain and apathy, which may make you feel unmotivated to change these habits. Constant sitting and eating can result in obesity, which is very difficult on the organs, bones, and entire body.
- High cholesterol
- Cataracts
- Diabetes

If you have any of these conditions, your Ayurvedic specialist will want to know how long you've had them, what you are doing about them, and if there is a history of these conditions in your family. She and your doctor will help you, taking all things about you and your history into consideration. If you don't show signs of these, but you have a lot of kapha in your constitution and a family history, these are conditions you may want to be aware of so you can be proactive by keeping your kapha in check. Keeping your doshas balanced by eating well, getting exercise, and having fun in your life is a great start.

Enjoy Kapha in Balance

Kapha in balance gives the world cohesion, compassion, nurturance, stability, moisture, calm, and sensuality. Kapha in balance shows up as kindness, calm, and compassion.

Your Ultimate Goal: Coming Into Balance

To achieve a state of balance among the doshas, which leads to health, these are the three principles you'll keep in mind:

1. Your state of being and everything you see, touch, taste, hear, and feel can be described in terms of qualities listed in the table.
2. Like increases like.
3. Opposites balance.

Creating health in Ayurveda means creating balance. You will be able to adjust your diet, type of exercise, and other factors in your life that can help you stay in balance throughout the various times of day, various seasons, and various times of life. Being in balance supports your biological functions, your psychological equilibrium, and your youthful spirit.

When the rishis realized Ayurveda, they realized that all life is connected, and that health is based on recognizing this wholeness and interconnectedness. Your health is based on your recognition that you are a whole being—body, mind, and spirit—and that your existence is in relationship to all that is.

According to Ayurveda you are both an individual and also a part of the entire fabric of existence. The way the elements were arranged in you at your conception makes you unique and individual. The precise choices you will make to balance yourself will differ from what your parents, your friends, and your children need to do for balance. At the same time, you and your loved ones are all part of the same fabric of life. You, the sun, the moon, the flowers, the earth, your animal friends, and all beings are exchanging the same energy.

2

The Benefits of Ayurveda

A Natural Way to Health and Joy

Just as trees, plants, and flowers are part of the natural world, so are you. The principles of the elements ether, air, fire, water, and earth are always at work inside of you and around you. As seasons change, as the time of day changes, and as years go by, your health depends on your ability to go with the natural flow of life. You and the natural world are in a constant relationship. Ayurveda as a medical science is based upon this practical, real, and exquisite foundation.

Ayurvedic Recommendations Are Natural

The herbs, oil, and food suggested by Ayurvedic practitioners are made of all-natural ingredients. Unlike drugs that are prescribed as part of allopathic medicine, the regimens and herbs that make up the Ayurvedic lifestyle do not cause side effects. Using Ayurveda is a natural and safe way to improve your health and your relationship to the life you're living.

Ayurveda also recognizes that your energy and thoughts toward the food you buy, prepare, and eat is as important as choosing the right ingredients. In other words, as you go shopping, as you cook, and as you eat, take time to appreciate the hard work and dedication of those who have made it possible for you to have this food. And if you grow your own herbs and food, you'll really notice your close relationship to what you are eating. Fill the food and the process of preparing it with your heartfelt care and love, and that energy will enhance the vital energy of the food. Also, get the freshest products you can find and afford.

Following Natural Cycles of Life

You may have noticed the many cycles of life. The moon has phases: new to full to new. The seasons cycle: spring, summer, fall, winter, spring. The sun rises, sets, and rises, and the days get shorter and longer as seasons cycle. There is a cycle of life as well, from childhood to young adulthood to the later years of life and then death. According to the tradition in India, where Ayurveda originates, birth-death-birth is also a cycle. After death, there is rebirth, and the cycle begins again. Just as there isn't a beginning and end to the way we see the sun rise and set and rise, there isn't a beginning or an end to life: Life follows a cycle.

Ayurveda recognizes that as the seasons cycle, you are affected. And as you go through your cycle of life, your needs change. Ayurveda teaches about the qualities of the seasons of nature and of life, and it offers ways to stay in balance through these changes. There's a way to both gently give in to the special attributes of each season while also making sure you stay in balance. This is how you'll remain healthy. For example, when the weather becomes cold and dry in winter, it affects you beyond a sense of physical discomfort. Winter is characterized as a vata time of year, and vata is associated with cold, dry, and mobile. In winter, the cold and dry air penetrates the skin, and it will affect bones, organs, muscles, and your body's biochemical processes if you don't add warmth and moisture to your body. For balancing the qualities of vata, particularly at this time of year, Ayurveda offers natural, simple, and logical recommendations for lifestyle and diet to help warm you up and pacify the effects that winter could otherwise have on your physical and mental health.

Once you learn about your constitution and the qualities attributed to each season, you will be able to live in harmony with the natural rhythms of life. That way, you can remain healthy, comfortable, and immune to disease throughout the year.

Daily Cycles

Just as there is a seasonal cycle, there is a daily cycle. While temperature and the number of hours of sunlight will vary throughout the year and throughout the world, there is a natural daily cycle that remains the same. Instead of trying to plan your activities and routine in conflict with the daily cycle, it's best for your overall health if you work with the natural cycles of vata, pitta, kapha as they occur each day.

The Daily Dosha Clock

Time of Day	Associated Dosha
6 a.m.–10 a.m.	kapha
10 a.m.–2 p.m.	pitta
2 p.m.–6 p.m.	vata
6 p.m.–10 p.m.	kapha
10 p.m.–2 a.m.	pitta
2 a.m.–6 a.m.	vata

The daily cycle helps you understand when it's best to wake up (before kapha time), when to eat your biggest meal (lunchtime, pitta time), and what time to go to sleep (before pitta time) based on the qualities associated with each dosha.

Ayurveda Provides a Whole System of Health

When you exhibit symptoms of imbalance or disease, Ayurveda takes into consideration your mental, physical, and energetic/spiritual state. For example, if you have a headache, Ayurveda doesn't just look at what could be causing this from a physical perspective. Ayurveda is interested in your entire lifestyle and diet, even if the symptom seems to be clearly a headache. This is because all aspects of you are connected. Your body, mind, and energy system are connected. Disease that begins in the mind or energy body, if not addressed, spreads to the physical body. Disease in the physical body affects the mind and spirit. For this reason, Ayurveda as a whole system of health examines your lifestyle, your diet, your stress levels, your environment, and your relationships to create harmony and balance.

AYURVEDA AS PREVENTIVE MEDICINE

Ayurvedic practices are ways to take care of yourself so you don't get sick. As preventive medicine, Ayurveda is a way to maintain health. When you follow the wisdom of Ayurveda, you are maintaining your health on a daily basis; nourishing your mind, body, and spirit; and creating the conditions for an easeful transition into the later years of your life. You do this by noticing early signs of imbalance, and taking the natural methods prescribed by Ayurveda to create equilibrium.

Using Ayurveda As Complementary Medicine

Ayurveda is a system of health that stands on its own, as a way of life. Because it is all natural and supports all of you—mind, body, and spirit—it can be used also as a complementary medicine. That means you can combine its practices with allopathic, or traditional, medicine.

IMPORTANT HEALTH NOTE

Ayurvedic herbs can interact with allopathic drugs. If you are seeing a Western medical doctor now, do not stop seeing her if you want to begin to talk to an Ayurvedic practitioner. Ease into Ayurveda. Continue with your medical doctor, then meet with an Ayurvedic specialist or Vaidya (Ayurvedic doctor) to see where she may be able to help. Always make sure that each doctor you talk to is aware of everything you're doing for your health.

Complementary Therapies

In combination with your allopathic treatments, your Ayurvedic practitioner may recommend any of a variety of what Western medicine calls complementary or alternative therapies. These therapies are called "complementary" because to traditional doctors, they are used as a complement to their prescriptions—not instead of what they prescribe. They are called "alternative" when they are used instead of allopathic medicine.

The following therapies are among those which your Ayurvedic practitioner may recommend. These therapies are all natural, have been used for thousands of years, and are used to restore your body by helping to circulate blood and lymph, support digestion, and boost immunity.

THERAPIES USED IN AYURVEDA

- **Aromatherapy:** using scents to pacify—or stimulate—the body and mind
- **Bodywork:** massaging herbalized oil over the entire body in rhythmic strokes
- **Marma therapy:** applying pressure to specific points on the body to help energy flow
- **Mindfulness practice:** becoming aware of what you are experiencing in each moment, which allows digestion, sleep, and other important physical and mental functions to occur naturally and easefully
- **Yoga, meditation, and pranayama:** cultivating mental equilibrium; promoting energy flow throughout the body; and enhancing physical strength, stamina, and health
- **Healing modalities with metals, gemstones, and colors:** using the energetic vibration of metals, gemstones, and colors to positively affect your energy system and overall health
- **Herbal supplements:** ingesting natural, whole herbs and spices in powder, liquid, or capsule form to enhance the body's ability to detoxify, absorb nutrients, and regain equilibrium

Many people choose to follow Ayurveda because it's preventive and picks up where traditional medicine leaves off. It treats the person for all of who she is, and supports her in creating a sustainable lifestyle for a lifetime of perfect health. It can also be used as a support for the body and mind when surgery or drugs are necessary.

Choosing Your Primary Care Doctor

If you are interested in natural ways of cultivating and maintaining health, you can find a doctor who practices integrative medicine. This means that she has been trained in allopathic medicine and has studied alternative therapies. This type of doctor might be very comfortable using a combination of allopathic treatments plus Ayurvedic recommendations to support your health in an ongoing way and during emergencies. An integrative doctor may not know a lot about Ayurveda, though she would recognize true healing takes into consideration mind, body, and energy, so she would likely support you seeing an Ayurvedic specialist for specific advice.

Self-Empowerment for Health and Longevity

Once you understand the basics of Ayurveda, you have the potential for less confusion and less frustration when you are faced with early signs of imbalance, the precursor to disease. Early signs of imbalance include such familiar conditions as: headache, constipation, sore throat, and irritability. When these types of early signs arise, Ayurveda tells you what immediate choices you can make that will support your immune system. You can turn to Ayurveda for guidance and natural recipes with herbs, teas, and spices that you can stock in your own kitchen.

It Just Makes Sense

Ayurveda demystifies the mystery of creating health. Those who don't gravitate toward science or aren't doctors may feel disconnected from any understanding of how to cultivate health. You may feel unable to understand what the body is, how it works, and how to work with it. Ayurveda doesn't require you to have an advanced biological or chemical understanding of the body. Instead, Ayurveda asks you to evaluate your health in terms of simple attributes. These are: dry, oily, light, heavy, cold, hot, unctuous (slimy), rough, soft, hard, subtle, gross, mobile, static, clear, cloudy, slow, sharp, dense, and liquid.

Notice How You Feel

Keep tabs on yourself and on your family. The sooner you notice signs of imbalance, the faster and easier it will be to correct them. The following are some questions to practice asking yourself. Practice noticing how you feel.

- How do you feel physically throughout your body?
- How is your energy level throughout the day?
- How do you feel when you interact with others?
- What is your sleeping pattern: how long, light or heavy, dreams, nightmares?
- Are you feeling happiness and joy in your life?
- How do you feel at work?
- How many times per day do you have bowel movements?
- How many times a day do you urinate?
- Do you make time for relaxation?
- Are you completing important tasks?

As you read farther into this book, you will become familiar with what your answers to those questions will tell you about your health. And you will learn and understand how to make adjustments in your lifestyle and diet when you notice imbalance. You will notice that by observing, nourishing, and nurturing yourself you will create the conditions for your body to heal itself.

COOK WITH YOUR CHILDREN

Because the energy you put into your food enhances its nourishing properties, see if you can make it a fun, loving, and special experience to cook with your children. Allow them to be part of an aspect of preparing a meal, or see if it works for them to help by adding in spices. Lead them to put loving intentions into the spices before tossing them in. Explain to them what the foods are, how they are grown, and how they nourish the body and mind. Notice the colors, textures, and scents. Enjoy the preparation process together.

When you talk to your Ayurvedic specialist, if you don't understand why she recommends things that she does, then ask her why. Understand what you're doing for your health, so you can continue to be an active participant in your wellness. With knowledge and understanding comes the ability to prevent disease from happening, or from getting worse if it's already begun.

Keeping Your Family Healthy

Ayurveda isn't a medical system that you only turn to when someone gets sick. Because it's about your lifestyle, it's for the whole family. If you use Ayurveda for yourself and for your children, you will notice a more balanced household with less irritability and illness. When you aren't spending energy treating illness, there is time for the fun and educational things in life: family time, playdates, school, exercise, and other activities you'd choose for your family.

Dynamic Approach to Overall Well-Being

As you change and as seasons change, your needs will change. The beauty of Ayurveda is that the advice it offers will feel natural to you. For example, in the summertime, especially if you are someone who has a good amount of pitta (the fire element), Ayurveda recommends cooling activities for the body such as swimming (during the cooler hours of the day). Most of us feel better with consistency, and because nature is always moving in cycles and we are changing, too, we need to learn to manage our emotions and stress that arise from all this uncertainty and flux. Ayurvedic practices help us do just that.

The Benefits of Allowing Emotions Instead of Repressing

Because of the various to-dos in life and because of a variety of other reasons, you may find yourself repressing emotions and/or repressing certain bodily functions. In other words, what if you have a really busy week at work? You might not only repress feelings that you have so that you can get through the workweek, but you also might even repress urges to go to the bathroom because you are just too busy.

When emotions come up, give them space. If you're at work when emotions want to break through and you can't take a break, make time when you get home to allow the emotions. Feel them fully; breathe deeply in and out several times until the emotions eventually dissipate. You can think of the metaphor of riding waves. Be the surfer, who rides them without getting swept away by them. It could take some time for the sensations of the emotion to rise up and then float away. When you allow yourself to feel the emotions, they can pass through you. If you repress them, you carry them within the very cells of your body.

DON'T REPRESS BODILY FUNCTIONS
Repressing is unhealthy for the mind and body. When it comes to elimination, make time for elimination first thing in the morning. And listen to your body when it's ready to eliminate because that's its way of clearing the waste out of your body to keep you healthy.

You may be repressing emotions for any number of reasons, so talking to a therapist, friends, and your doctors and healers about what you are experiencing is important. In addition, all aspects of your life contribute to how you will experience the emotions. What you eat, if you exercise, how well you sleep, and more contribute to your reactions to life and to your own emotions when they come up. Ayurveda is dynamic because your emotions and state of mind will shift, and Ayurveda can be there to support you with guidance for what to do when you experience different states of mind.

Find Time and Ways for Relaxation

When you become stressed-out and overwhelmed, your body kicks in to fight-or-flight response. Your heart beats faster, your breath becomes shallow, and you may become tense. The body is not meant to stay in fight-or-flight mode. Fight-or-flight is meant for emergencies. The body needs periods in the relaxation response, during which it will perform its normal functions. Your mind needs periods of rest, too, which you can give it through meditation, breathing exercises, yoga, and visualizations.

The more relaxation time you can bring to your body, mind, and spirit, the more you will be able to make clear decisions in your life, enjoy physical health, and age well. Ayurveda gives you practical, simple, and effective ways to enhance your quality of life, which you will learn in the following chapters. And though this will require some lifestyle and dietary changes, as you adopt an Ayurvedic lifestyle, you could actually enjoy yourself!

PART II

50 Exercises for Balance

3

Lifestyle and Routine

Create Conditions for Balance Each Morning

Ayurveda provides you with a nourishing paradigm for starting off your day, so begin to connect to the rhythm of the natural world the moment you wake up. Can you imagine how your day might feel different if you were to take some time to smoothly transition from sleep to wakefulness first thing in the morning? Many people are so lethargic that they can't get out of bed, and when they eventually do get out of bed, their day starts off slowly and sluggishly. Ayurveda recommends a morning routine to help you start your day off from a good place.

> **MANAGING A MORNING TRANSITION WITH KIDS**
> If somehow you can get up twenty minutes earlier than the rest of the family to do at least some parts of the routine for yourself, that would be wonderful. If not, these routines are also helpful for children (in modified form, depending on their ages—talk to your Ayurvedic specialist about it), so let them join in!

The Importance of the Transition

After being asleep for seven to nine hours (the ideal amount of time to sleep), your body and mind need a little space and care so they are ready for the big day ahead. If you don't take some time to transition, you're not listening to what your body and mind need.

Ayurveda teaches a nurturing and balancing way to transition from your nighttime stillness to morning activity. By doing this you create a smooth transition from sleep to activity, integrating the benefits of your sleep and creating a good foundation for your day. After your morning routine, you are ready to go from a place of centered groundedness. The morning routine also supports the flow of bodily fluids (such as blood and lymph), builds immunity, creates mental stability, prepares the body for movement, and much more.

Because everyone is so busy nowadays, people have become distanced from nature and the needs of the mind and body. This disassociation from your needs, and from nature's rhythm, leads to imbalance and disease. Keeping up this daily nourishing morning routine is a good form of self-discipline designed to take time for yourself. You'll feel real health benefits if you are consistent.

This morning routine is focused on cleaning out your sense organs and assisting in the elimination of toxins after your body has performed digestion in the middle of the night. You'll be starting your day clean, fresh, and with the intention for balance.

HOW TO DO THE MORNING ROUTINE

1. **Scraping the Tongue.** This will clear the *ama* (undigested substances) off of your tongue. Use a metal tongue scraper, and carefully swipe it across the tongue until you've rid the tongue of ama. In between swipes, rinse the scraper off under warm water.

2. **Neti Pot and Nasal Oil.** This part of your routine will keep the nasal passages clean and moist, which will keep bacteria and other foreign particles from settling into your body's system. To do this, buy a ceramic neti pot, and follow the instructions. You will need warm sterile water and noniodized sea salt. After using the neti pot, carefully tilt your head from side to side over the sink so all the water comes out. Then, use nasya (or sesame) oil. To do this, lean your head back, and drip a few drops of oil into your right nostril. Keep your head back for about thirty seconds and massage the oil into the nose. It's okay if some slides down your throat. Bring your head to a neutral position for a moment. Then, tilt your head back and repeat the steps on the other side by dropping oil into your left nostril. Once on each side, each morning.

3. **Oil in the Ears.** Place sesame oil on your fingers and gently and carefully rub the inside and the outside of each ear. Be sure to massage the ear lobe too.

4. **Rosewater Spray in Your Eyes.** This keeps your eyes moist and clear. It's especially helpful during allergy season.

5. **Self-Massage with Oil.** If you are primarily vata or kapha, use warm sesame oil. If you want to pacify pitta, use coconut oil. Begin your self-massage by massaging your arms. Use long, steady strokes on the long bones, and use a circular motion to massage oil into the joints. Do the same for your legs. Continue to massage every part of your body, giving it loving, soothing attention. The oil will sink into the skin, and lubricate deep tissues. You can also oil your head. The oil will come out of your hair if you use shampoo. You can shower after you give yourself a massage, then tap your skin with a towel before getting dressed so the oil doesn't get on your clothing.

6. **A Glass of Warm Water.** A glass of warm water in the morning can help with your morning elimination. It's very healthy to go to the bathroom first thing in the morning, each day.

7. **Joint Warm-Ups and a Few Gentle Yoga Postures.** This will prepare the body for the movements you'll be doing throughout your day. This easeful physical activity can also help with your morning elimination and help ground you in the present moment.

8. **A Walk Outside.** Even if you walk for just a short distance, going outside connects you to the freshness of the morning's air. It can help you wake up and feel the qualities of the elements supporting you.

9. **Pranayama.** You can choose a pranayama that suits your own constitution and how you are feeling today. If you are exhibiting signs of imbalanced vata, choose a pranayama for calming and grounding. If you are kaphic, start with some deep breaths and then choose a warming breath. If you are predominantly showing signs of pitta imbalance, choose a pitta-pacifying breath.

The morning routine allows you to start your day from a clean, fresh, and healthy place. It supports your immune system and prepares your mind and body for the activity and work that you'll be doing the rest of the day. It's so supportive to your health to make a smooth and mindful transition into your day.

Follow Nature's Clock

The natural clock has the qualities of the doshas, just as you do. The hours between 2 a.m. and 6 a.m. is vata time; 6 a.m. to 10 a.m. is kapha time; 10 a.m. to 2 p.m. is pitta time; 2 to 6 p.m. is vata time; 6 to 10 p.m. is kapha time; 10 p.m. to 2 a.m. is pitta time. During these times you are affected by those qualities. When your constitution is the same as the time of day, then those qualities will be heightened for you. Everyone is affected by nature's clock, however, and so there are general guidelines of when to wake up, have your heaviest meal, and go to bed *(see image on page 3 of the insert)*.

Keeping a Schedule

Waking up naturally is best. Allowing natural light to come into your bedroom so you wake up to it keeps you in sync with nature. Ayurveda recommends you get up before 6 a.m. (or sunrise) so that you aren't waking up during kapha time.

Kapha time, 6 a.m.–10 a.m., is a great time to be doing your morning routine because the earth and water qualities of kapha support lubrication of the joints and movement. If you are predominantly kapha, it will be supportive to you to include some kind of activity in the morning (between 6 a.m. and 8 a.m.), such as *asanas* (yoga poses) or a brisk walk or run before you have breakfast. Eat a light breakfast around 8 a.m., and then begin work around 9 a.m. For pitta, start with a calming morning routine, and do asanas or run before breakfast. Eat breakfast around 7 or 8 a.m., and then begin your regular work activities around 9 a.m. after eating a leisurely breakfast. If you are predominantly vata, keep the entire morning calm as you do your routine, and eat your breakfast slowly. Begin your workday around 10 a.m.

After kapha time is pitta time. It's best to eat your heaviest meal at lunchtime, when nature has pitta qualities. For all doshas this is the time to eat the heaviest meal. If you are predominantly pitta, be mindful of your interactions with others and the activities you do between 10 a.m. and 2 p.m. This is when your fiery qualities can be most aggravated by the time of day.

Vata time is 2 p.m.–6 p.m. For pitta and kapha types, this is a great time to be engaged in work and mental activities. If you are primarily vata, be mindful during these hours. Do what you need to feel grounded. You may need to take breaks from work at this time. Take time to meditate. If you can, take a nap. Drink some hot tea. Take time to relax during these hours.

Kapha time is 6 p.m.–10 p.m. This is the perfect time to have a leisurely dinner. Begin to unwind from the day. Allow the kapha energy to ground you and prepare you for bedtime. For all types, it's best to go to sleep by or around 10 p.m., while still in kapha time.

Practice Mindfulness for Balance

Mindfulness refers to bringing your awareness to the present moment. It means paying attention to what you're doing, how you're doing it, and what's going on around you in each moment. When you're in the present moment, you can enjoy the peace of being "right here, right now," where regrets about past events or concerns about future possibilities won't cause you stress.

When your awareness is in on the present moment, you can deal with what comes up more effectively, and your physical body can relax and perform its vital functions. Otherwise, when you are stressed-out, your body goes into fight-or-flight mode (also called a sympathetic response): Your breath becomes shallow, your heart rate increases, and many other "emergency" responses are triggered in the body. This obstructs the free and natural flow of energy in the body. So, you want to engage a parasympathetic response (also called a relaxation response). Keeping your mind at peace through mindfulness is one technique that will help.

Why Be Mindful?

When you're being mindful, you are able to enjoy, appreciate, and benefit from what's going on in your life in a vivid way. It means you're not primarily living in the past or in the future. Time can actually feel stretched when you live this way, and you will more thoroughly experience life. For example, when you mindfully eat—when you chew slowly, savor the tastes, and pay attention to the fact that you are eating—you will feel full after eating less than you would eat if you weren't being mindful; your body will be more powerfully affected by the experience of eating; and you'll likely remember later in the day that you've eaten.

Being mindful also means checking in with yourself to see how you are doing. When you don't check in with yourself and pay attention to your mental, emotional, and physical states, you can unknowingly start accumulating mental, emotional, and energetic debris. When you don't digest it and clear it out, then it throws you off balance. The longer you are out of balance, and the more debris you hold on to, the more your overall health becomes compromised. According to Ayurveda, physical symptoms are often a result of what you experience in life and how you digest it energetically, mentally, and physically.

A Mindfulness Exercise

The more you practice being mindful, the more often you will start to live that way, sometimes without consciously thinking about doing it. Here's an exercise you can do as often as you like.

1. When you can remember, at any point in your day, stop what you are doing for a moment.
2. With your eyes closed deepen your breath, and send your awareness to the various parts of your body, starting with the top of your head and moving downward to the feet.
3. As you send awareness to each body part, inhale and imagine sending prana to that body part. Exhale, and imagine releasing stress.
4. After you've brought your awareness down to the feet, notice if anywhere in the body you feel discomfort. Make small movements of the body to release tension and stiffness.
5. Finally, take a few very deep inhalations and exhalations. On the final exhalation, bring a small smile to your lips.
6. Open your eyes and take another moment to appreciate that break.

You can take mindfulness breaks like this throughout your day; however, you don't have to take a break to practice mindfulness. You can bring mindfulness to any activity. It simply means being present with what is and being intentional about what you're doing. It might sound simple, but in fact it's surprising how often the mind isn't on what's happening right in the present moment.

Engage in Nourishing Bodywork

Bodywork is an important part of Ayurvedic healthy living. The treatments facilitate the flow of energy, blood, and lymph throughout the body. They also balance the doshas, and each has additional benefits depending on what you need. Some types of treatments and oils will stimulate energy; others will primarily calm the nervous system.

- *Abhyanga* is the application of oil to your entire body. The Ayurvedic bodyworker warms oil infused with herbs specifically selected for you. Then she applies the oil to your body in a way that supports physical and energetic circulation, loosens toxins, and relaxes the mind. It's also called Abhyanga when you give yourself an Ayurvedic oil massage.
- *Abhyanga-Gharshana* includes a silk-glove massage before the Abhyanga treatment. The silk-glove massage cleans the skin and stimulates circulation, before the oil sinks in to nourish your body.
- *Vishesh* is a treatment of oil infused with herbs applied to the body in rapid, rhythmic movements. This helps facilitate energetic, arterial, and lymphatic flow throughout the body.
- *Shirodhara* is a steady stream of warm, herbalized oil poured onto the forehead, balancing and calming the mind.

Often Ayurvedic bodyworkers will combine treatments. For example, you could request Abhyanga-Shirodhara. To find a trained practitioner near you, look for Ayurvedic specialists in your area who can do the bodywork or who can recommend where to have it done. Also, some spas and retreat centers are now offering Ayurvedic treatments, chakra balancing, and other therapies that balance your energy and support the body.

Tune In to Your Chakras

Chakra simply means "wheel" or "disc," and the seven major chakras in your body are spinning energy wheels where energy pathways converge. You have other chakras in the body, and beyond the body in your energy field. The ancient rishis discovered that by meditating on the seven major chakras in ascending order, they could awaken and move energy through their physical and energetic bodies. It was through this type of meditation that they would reach liberation or enlightenment.

How Balancing Chakras Balances You

Beginning thousands of years ago, rishis and their students meditated on the seven chakras as a path to clearing karma and reaching enlightenment. Chakra theory came to the West in the early twentieth century, and Theosophists took great interest. Their discoveries further illuminate the connection between how freely energy flows in the body and how healthy and youthful a person is.

When the chakras are balanced, it means that energy is flowing in the body in a way that is neither too fast nor too slow. It means that you are firing on all cylinders. Your mind and body are being fed with just the right amount of life-force energy, or prana, to keep you functioning with optimum clarity, ease, contentment, and focus.

When any of the chakras is out of balance, it's spinning too sluggishly or too quickly. What affects the chakras' ability to function are the same factors that affect your overall health: your lifestyle, your emotional and mental state, and how you're treating your physical body through diet, movement, and stress management. Your health has a symbiotic relationship with the health of the chakras. If you are feeling unbalanced it can throw them off balance, and if they are out of balance it will cause you to be off balance.

Chakras and the Elements

The chakras each have a stem in the spine, and they flower out into the body. In the following table, you will see the name of each chakra, its general placement that you can use for beginning visualizations, and the element that it's linked to *(see image on page 4 of the insert).*

Chakra	Placement	Element	Color
Root (Muladhara)	perineum/tailbone	earth	red
Sacrum (Svadhisthana)	lower abdomen	water	orange
Solar Plexus (Manipura)	just above the navel	fire	yellow
Heart (Anahata)	center of breastbone	air	green
Throat (Vishuddha)	base of neck	ether	blue
Third Eye (Ajna)	between the two eyes on the forehead	mind	indigo
Crown (Sahasrara)	top of the head	consciousness	white, purple, or gold

Identifying chakras in this way with the elements, you can get a sense of how they are connected to the doshas.

Chakras and the Doshas

Use the elements as the unifying factor between the chakras and the doshas to help you understand how to use chakra healing to balance the doshas.

For example, if you're feeling ungrounded that is a sign of vata imbalance. So, you want to bring energy to the chakras that will help you feel grounded. The first chakra is of the earth element; it is grounding. The second chakra is of water, which is also balancing for vata. The third chakra is fire, heating. So, if you're feeling excess vata, you need to bring more energy to those lower chakras to help you feel grounded.

Pitta can be related to the solar plexus chakra and third eye (fire, intellect, and connection to wisdom). With pitta as predominant, you may feel disconnected from the subtle, profound energies associated with the heart and throat chakras. When it comes to these chakras, you will be a good public speaker and advocate, but perhaps you will have trouble with true connection and good, comfortable communication in personal and intimate relationships.

Kapha energy can be linked to the root and sacral chakras. If you're predominantly kapha, you may not have a strong manipura chakra, which will affect your digestive fire as well as your self-esteem. Bring some of that energy up from the root and sacral chakras to energize the manipura and higher chakras.

Simple Chakra Healing Exercise

There are several resources available to learn various simple, engaging, and practical chakra healing methods that you can do in your own home, with your children, or by yourself. Here is one simple method for bringing energy to the various chakras.

Visualizing the color associated with each chakra is one way to energize that chakra. When you would like to bring energy to a particular chakra, envision the corresponding color glowing brightly in the area of that chakra. Try this visualization:

1. Sit with your sitting bones rooted into the chair or earth.
2. Elongate the spine so you are sitting up straight, and the crown of your head is pointing toward the ceiling.
3. Relax the jaw, relax the arms, relax the belly.
4. Deepen your inhalations and exhalations.
5. On an inhalation envision drawing the color red in through your nostrils and way down deep into the perineum.
6. On the exhalation, exhale slowly, imagining any muddy color leaving the body.

7. Repeat this two more times, envisioning the color red going into the region of the perineum.

8. Do this same visualization at each chakra, with its corresponding color. Inhale that color deep into the appropriate area, and exhale any unwanted energy.

9. When you get to the crown chakra, on your final exhalation, return to normal breathing.

10. Breathe normally for a few moments, noticing the effects of the visualization. Then, open your eyes.

This is a visualization you can do for all the chakras. Even if it seems that just one chakra is out of balance, it always is helpful to give attention to each chakra because all chakras do affect each other.

Use Balancing Aromas

Aromas are helpful tools for balancing the doshas. Each time you make yourself a meal, remember this is a chance to fill your kitchen with aromas. For example, if you're in the mood for an apple, cook the apple in honey, and don't forget to sprinkle it with at least one spice, such as cinnamon. Experiment with the various aromas, learning which scents affect you in positive ways. Since everyone is unique, you will have your preference.

What Are Essential Oils?

Essential oils are all natural and used for a variety of conditions and ailments. They are concentrated oils that come from trees, plants, and grasses. Their aromas carry the healing properties and energy from their original source and can be used in baths, lotions, and oils, and in diffusers.

Essential oils are not meant to be put directly onto the skin. You can mix essential oils in high-quality oil such as extra-virgin, cold-pressed olive oil, or sesame oil, and then put a few drops of that mixture into your bath or onto your skin. The typical way to figure out the ratio of base oil to essential oil is to measure the base oil in milliliters, then divide that number in half. That number is the maximum number of drops of essential oil you'll need to add to the mix. It doesn't take much; essential oils are very potent.

For Vata

- **Cooking:** In general, cooking with cardamom, cinnamon, ginger, nutmeg, and clove could be beneficial to vata.
- **Bath or Massage Oil:** Aromas that are balancing for vata are pine, lavender, and frankincense. Red rose, musk, and camphor, because of their sweet and warming tones, can also balance vata.

For Pitta

- **Cooking:** Mint, fennel, and cammomile.
- **Bath or Massage Oil:** Aromas that balance pitta have the opposite qualities of pitta, so the scents will be sweet, cooling, and calming. Rose, lemongrass, peppermint, gardenia, sandalwood, and jasmine are specific scents to test out and see which you like the best.
- **Aromas Before Bedtime:** Pitta dreams can be violent. Using aromatherapy earlier in the day and before bedtime can help calm the mind. Lavender is often used in bedrooms, bathrooms, and spas to soothe anxiety and an overactive mind. Try using a lavender spray in your room, lavender in your diffuser, or a lavender-scented candle (blow out the candle before falling asleep).

For Kapha

- **Cooking:** Cinnamon, thyme, basil, and rosemary.
- **Bath or Massage Oil:** You'll want to go for what is stimulating and warming when you want to balance kapha. Avoid aromas that are sweet or cooling. Aromas to try in diffusers and oils for kapha are: camphor, musk, myrrh, and sage. Remember that the best oil to use as a base oil for kapha is corn oil. Because kaphas don't necessarily need more oil on the body or in a bath, you could skip the oil altogether and use a diffuser when you want to use aromatherapy. Another alternative to using a diffuser is to burn sage in a bunch—sage is often bound together to be used for smudging, so it's already bound together for you.

ROSEWATER SPRAY

There is a type of Ayurvedic rosewater spray that can be sprayed into the eyes to cool them and reduce redness. This spray is refreshing for all types, especially pitta, because it's cooling, and the scent of rose is sweet. Rose also acts as an anti-inflammatory to help reduce puffiness. Keep a bottle at home and another at the office to use after staring at the computer screen too long.

Help Your Children Balance Themselves

No two children (in fact, no two people) are the same. Using Ayurveda as your guide, you'll be able to evaluate how your children look, act, feel, and digest their food, so you can determine how to help them stay healthy. Ayurveda will help you account for the individual needs of each person to create health, harmony, and happiness in the home.

Vata

A great help for vata is to create routine. Try to make the mornings the same and predictable for yourself and your family. During the school week, have breakfast at the same time, and have dinner at the same time each day when you can (around their extracurricular activities). Expect your children to go to bed at the same time each night (when possible), and have a bedtime routine. A bedtime routine for you (and your children) could look like this:

1. Turn off the television, computers, and cell phones an hour before bedtime.
2. Go outside for at least five minutes and get grounded and calm. Observe the moonlight, stars, and the nighttime sounds together. Everyone, take nice, soothing long breaths. Let go of the day.
3. Come inside, and slowly enjoy a cup of warm spiced milk.
4. Brush teeth and get dressed for bed, with as much calm and peacefulness as possible.
5. Get into bed, and before falling asleep enjoy sinking into the support of the bed. Take a few breaths, let go of the day even more, and think of at least one thing you're grateful for.

Having a nighttime routine will help you stay mindful of the transition from activity to sleep, and can help children and adults alike feel secure and grounded.

Pitta

There's so much you can do for your children to keep their pitta in balance. If you have a child who is predominantly pitta, add practices into her life that will balance pitta's qualities and that she will be able to continue when she is older (especially in the pitta time of her life). You can disguise pitta-pacifying things as fun, cooling activities and special family-time excursions for you and your children.

Being able to get all As in school, play first base on the baseball team, and be the star in the school play every year are ways that pitta types may be able to gain supportive recognition. Bright and capable children will work hard, especially when they are encouraged and rewarded for their achievements. They may get rewards, such as: getting into the best schools, attending the best universities, and getting jobs in fields they are passionate about.

The important thing to recognize if your child is predominantly pitta is to see if those qualities are not being balanced. So ask yourself these questions:

○ Does my child get in arguments at school?
○ Does my child have digestive issues, like acid reflux, diarrhea, or vomiting?
○ Does my child have severe acne, rash, or other skin inflammations?
○ Is my child's mood characterized by being irritated and angered at home?
○ Is my child very uncomfortable in the heat?
○ Did my daughter start her period early?
○ Does my child stay up past midnight, reading?
○ Is my child really competitive in sports, with grades, and with my other children?

If you answer "yes" to these questions about your child's temperament and appearance, it would be a great help to your child's health, life experience, and eventual aging process if you would help her balance pitta through diet and creating a pitta-pacifying environment at home. As usual that means creating an environment for that child that has the opposite qualities of her pitta qualities.

Kapha

The kapha years are your earliest years. Babies and children are in their kapha time. It's the time of life when healthy babies will be chubby, they will be attached to their mother, and they will be growing (which kapha supports). You will notice that children produce a lot of mucus, too, which is part of kapha's support of the growth process. As Ayurveda expert Dr. John Douillard said, "For kids, this lubrication is extremely significant because it supports their elastic growth—up to a foot each year. The amount of lubrication in a kid's body is one reason why a seven-year-old child can slide down a set of stairs laughing with each bump whereas an eighty-year-old would simply break."

As children are growing it's important to notice how their kapha is affecting them. For example, if the mucus production gets too high, and they are developing chronic colds, you will want to help balance out their kapha with the kapha balance tips for meals and activities.

If you notice your child is gaining weight, sleeps a lot, and has a high capacity for compassion, all of these are kapha qualities and consistent with this time of life. Because of this, your child will need your acceptance that these are the natural tendencies in this time of life, and you can help him stay in balance by helping provide the opposite qualities in food and lifestyle. This is a perfect time of life to teach him healthy eating and exercise habits—and exercise can mean playing sports, playing fun active games outside, and taking nice walks together.

Cultivate Self-Awareness and Compassion

Becoming aware of what you say, think, feel, and do is an essential part of healthy living. This is true for many reasons. At the very basic level, you must be able to observe yourself in order to know what's working, what's not working, and how to create balance. Practice noticing what you do, how you do it, and how that affects the way you experience health and your life. By observing yourself—your thoughts, your reactions, your energy levels, how you treat others, how you treat yourself, what you eat, what you do for exercise, how you feel about exercise, etc.—you can learn what's supporting your health and what's detracting from you being able to live a life that is naturally healthful and beautiful. Once you can notice how you are, Ayurveda can give you the tools and guidance you need.

AVOID NEGATIVE THOUGHTS

Thinking negative thoughts is just as unhealthy for you as eating unhealthy food. Negative emotions, thoughts, and feelings move from energetic dis-ease to mental and physical disease. It's just as important to learn new ways of working with your mental and energetic bodies as it is to learn new ways of taking care of your physical body.

When you observe yourself, practice observing with compassion. When you notice something about you that you think you want to change, notice it with compassion. For example, if you notice you don't eat well all day and then you are so hungry you eat a whole bag of candy, just notice that. Then, notice if your tendency is to want to mentally punish yourself, thinking you've done something "bad." See if you can turn that around. Instead of thinking you've done something wrong, ask yourself if you eat bags of candy often enough that it's a behavior you'd like to change. If so, that's a good thing to notice: This is something you would like to change. You have the power to do that, and you don't have to mentally punish yourself. Instead, educate yourself about what would be a healthier, more satisfying, and sweet snack.

It's important as a first step to notice the habits you want to change, have compassion for yourself, and then look to another way of doing things—such as Ayurveda.

How to Cultivate Compassion

You cannot feel compassion for others if you do not feel it for yourself. Any parts of yourself you reject, you will reject in others. Parts of yourself that you repress will trigger you when you see it in others. The more compassionate awareness you can have for all aspects of who you are, the more you can have that for others. Honest compassion for yourself and others is a recipe for personal and global healing.

To cultivate compassion for yourself, be gentle with yourself. Spend time in meditation allowing thoughts to arise so you can see what they are. When you meditate, you sit in stillness. As thoughts arise, notice that they are there. Compassionately notice whatever they are. And, then, allow them to drift by. Focus on your breath, the present moment of the breath flowing in and out without you needing to control it. As thoughts arise, again, notice them. Do not judge them. And then allow them to float by like the clouds in the sky. Compassionately acknowledge your thoughts, without judgment and without attaching to them during your meditation. This is a way to cultivate compassion for yourself.

Being compassionate doesn't mean you have to be friends with everyone you meet. It does mean that you'll do your best, even with someone you can't bear to spend time with, to honor the light that is in them. It doesn't mean you compromise your well-being by trying to fix or heal them. If you can't be friends with them, it's okay. You can acknowledge that to yourself, create a boundary by not spending time with the person, and still know he is suffering, or has suffered, and is doing his best in the world just as you are.

Metta Meditation

Another way to cultivate compassion is metta meditation. To do this, get in a comfortable, seated position as you would for seated meditation. Close your eyes and get grounded. Feel your sitting bones rooted into the cushion that you're seated on. Take a deep inhalation and a long exhalation. Do this deep breathing a few more times. Then, be still. Watch your breath for a few exhalations. Then, follow these steps, with an open heart:

1. Say this silently to yourself: "May I be happy. May I be healthy. May I be safe."

2. Call to mind someone whom you love dearly. Hold this person in your heart, and silently send this wish to that person: "May you be happy. May you be healthy. May you be safe."

3. Call to mind someone you don't know very well, whose path you cross now and then. Send this heartfelt wish silently to that person: "May you be happy. May you be healthy. May you be safe."

4. Call to mind everyone in your neighborhood, village, or city, and silently send this wish to them: "May you be happy. May you be healthy. May you be safe."

5. Call to mind someone with whom you have a conflict. Knowing he is suffering, silently send him this wish: "May you be happy. May you be healthy. May you be safe."

6. Call to mind all the service-minded people in the world, who in any way large or small serve others in their work or in their lives. Send them this wish: "May you be happy. May you be healthy. May you be safe."

7. Hold in your heart all beings everywhere, and send out this wish: "May you be happy. May you be healthy. May you be safe."

8. Take a moment in silence. Breathe. Notice how you feel. Acknowledge the meditative space you've been in and take a moment to transition back into your day.

Metta meditation helps you cultivate compassion for yourself first, and then give it out to the rest of the world. This practice helps you really feel and see that everyone and everything is connected and wants to be happy, healthy, and secure.

Ease Into Bedtime

Getting a good night's sleep is so important for your mental, physical, and energetic bodies. Modern medical studies show you need seven to nine hours of sleep to regulate your metabolism. As with all parts of your daily cycle it will help you and your nervous system if you transition mindfully from one phase to the next. So rather than work until late at night, and then conk out at bedtime from exhaustion and overwork, you could stop work earlier and have an easeful, nice transition from your working hours into your sleeping hours. Creating this sense of calm and ease, making space between work and sleep, gives your body the signal that there's plenty of time for rest and sleep.

Why Do You Stay Up Late?

Decide ahead of time what time you would like to go to sleep. Ayurveda recommends going to bed by or around 10 p.m. That might not be possible for you. Perhaps 11 p.m. is a more reasonable goal. Being intentional about your schedule helps create structure for important self-care routines.

Time to Unwind

Instead of watching TV or working late, what could you be doing for yourself and your health between the hours of 8 p.m.–10 p.m.? If you were to go to bed around 10 p.m., you would start unwinding around 7 p.m. or 8 p.m. That means, when it's 7 p.m. or 8 p.m., you stop engaging in work and stimulating activities. Have some soothing tea. Read a meditative or inspirational book. Give yourself an oil massage. Take a hot bath. Write a fun letter. Spend time with your family or your friends, not watching television or on the computer. Go for a night walk. Read poetry. Knit. For a couple of hours, give yourself nourishing, relaxing time. Then slip into bed by 10 p.m., without having the speedy work or Internet communication still buzzing around in your mind.

4

Breathwork

Learn the Importance of Proper Breathing

The purity of the air you breathe is, of course, very important. But how you breathe is equally if not more important. That's why breathwork is a key part of Ayurveda practice. There are important general guidelines for practicing breath control, or pranayama. Review this checklist every time you are going to practice pranayama.

- Pranayama should be practiced in a quiet, clean, and tranquil location with good ventilation.
- Pranayama should be practiced on an empty stomach.
- Pranayama should be done in a comfortable position, either on the floor or in a chair, with the spine, neck, and head erect. Clothing should be loose and comfortable. (Sometimes you may do pranayama while already in another yoga posture, if you already are experienced with pranayama.)
- Avoid strain with all pranayama practices. Do not practice pranayama during times of illness. If you experience negative side effects, physical or emotional, discontinue the practice and consult with a qualified yoga teacher or a physician.

When finished with your breathing practice, return to normal breathing for a minute or two, then lie down in Savasana (Corpse Pose) for several minutes to allow for integration.

$$\ast$$

Nadi Shodhana for
Vata Balance

When vata dosha goes out of balance, you may feel a heightened sense of indecisiveness, anxiety, and fear. Anxiety and fear tend to affect the breath by producing short, shallow upper-chest breathing. Thus, the most important breathing practices to tame vata dosha are those that produce a calm and steady breath pattern.

Understanding the Nadis

When speaking of the power of the breath, it's helpful to know about the nadi system. Nadis are the energy channels of the body that provide the "vehicle" for the flow of prana (life force) and consciousness throughout the entire body. The central nadi is called the Sushumna, which runs from the base or root of the spinal column (muladhara chakra) to the crown of the head (sahasrara chakra). Two other important nadis, the Ida and Pingala, begin at the base of the spine, crisscross over and around the Sushumna, and end up together in the nostrils. The chakras are energy vortexes (sometimes described as spinning wheels of energy) that exist where the Ida and Pingala cross.

The Ida ends at the left hemisphere of the brain (some say the left nostril), and the Pingala ends at the right. The Ida has cooling properties and relates to the feminine principle. The Pingala has heating properties and relates to the masculine principle.

Throughout the day the breath automatically fluctuates between the two nadis. There is a shift from right to left nostrils being open about every sixty to ninety minutes in the healthy person. This balancing of Ida and Pingala causes prana to flow evenly and is part of the natural balancing process of the body.

When the nadis are clear and balanced, certain external signs appear. They are lightness and leanness of the body, brilliancy in complexion, increased gastric fire, and the absence of restlessness in the body. These are some obvious signs of a healthy body.

INSTRUCTIONS FOR NADI SHODHANA

1. Sit comfortably with the spine straight.
2. Hold your right hand in Vishnu mudra (the hand position where the thumb, ring finger, and pinky are extended, and the other fingers are bent).
3. Close off the right nostril with the right thumb.
4. Softly breathe in through the left nostril.
5. At the top of that breath, close off the left nostril with the right ring finger and exhale through the right nostril.
6. At the bottom of that exhalation, breathe back in through the right nostril.
7. At the top of that inhalation, close off the right nostril with the right thumb and exhale out the left nostril.
8. Repeat this pattern for a minute or two, keeping the breath soft, regular, and steady, and the shoulders relaxed.

If your arm gets tired, you can prop it on a cushion or with your other hand. When the nadis are open, there is a natural feeling of calm and ease of being.

✳

Dirgha Breath, Lying on Your Back, for Vata Balance

Another important breath is Dirgha Breath, the three-part or yogic breath. When you do this, you welcome the breath deep into the lungs, causing the belly and ribs to expand three-dimensionally. An easy way to learn this is by lying on your back with the knees bent. Once in this position, follow these instructions:

1. Place your hands on the belly, pressing down slightly to give a bit of resistance as you breathe in.
2. Inhale deeply, so that the hands rise as you breathe in.
3. Simply relax and exhale. Practice this a while. Then rest.
4. Place your hands over the sides of your ribs. As you breathe in, try to make your ribs expand outward, into your hands. Imagine your sides having fish gills as you breathe through them.
5. Place one hand on the upper chest and collarbones and the other on the back side of your shoulders, just below the neck. As you inhale, try to breathe so deeply that even these two areas expand.
6. Combine all three aspects of this breath. Breathing in, belly, side ribs, and upper chest and back expand with the movement of the breath flowing into the lungs. Breathing out, empty out. Release and let go.

Practice Dirgha Breath for one to five minutes. Then pause and notice the effect. You will likely feel calmer and more grounded, awake and clear. That is, you will feel more "balanced." A major goal of Ayurveda is achieving that sense of a balanced state in body and mind.

✳

Warming Breath and
So Hum Steady Breath
for Vata Balance

The Warming Breath helps correct the cooling tendency of vata. The right nostril relates to the Pingala or sun energy side. Using the same hand position as in nadi shodhana, start by breathing in the right nostril and exhaling out the left. Repeat. Breathe back in the right and breathe out the left. Continue for a minute or so.

So Hum Steady Breath

This is a steady in-and-out breath, combined with the silent repetition of the words (mantra) *So* and *Hum*. The breath naturally makes these two sounds: *Sooooooo* as you inhale, and *Hummmmmm* as you exhale. This practice is very helpful in balancing the Ida and Pingala.

1. Place your hands over your ears and as you breathe in, silently say the word *so*. Let the "soooo" extend the full length of the in-breath.
2. As you breathe out, silently say the word *hum*, extending that sound for the full length of the exhalation.

Once you get the gist of this, continue the practice with your hands resting comfortably in your lap. And, remember, for all of these breathing practices, it is important to be seated comfortably, head aligned over the spine, with your back upright and shoulders relaxed.

Lunar Breath/Left Nostril Breath (Chandra Bhedana) for Pitta Balance

Lunar Breath helps to expel excess pitta. By directing the breath through the left nostril, which is associated with the cooling energy of the moon, the mind and body become soothed and relaxed. If you suffer from low blood pressure, depression, colds, flu, or any other respiratory conditions, avoid this pranayama. Follow these instructions:

1. Sit comfortably with a long spine.
2. Hold up your right hand and fold your index and middle fingers into the palm of your hand, keeping the thumb, ring finger, and pinky extended (Vishnu mudra).
3. Seal your right nostril with your thumb and take a slow and complete breath *in* through your left nostril.
4. Seal your left nostril with your ring finger, release your thumb, and exhale *out* of the right nostril.
5. Repeat this sequence—inhaling through your left nostril and exhaling through your right.
6. Continue for three to five minutes.

In addition to calming your mind and cooling your entire body, this breathing exercise relaxes your muscles, promotes tranquility, and increases introspection.

Cooling Breath (Shitali) for Pitta Balance

Cooling Breath is done by inhaling through your mouth and exhaling through your nose. This breathing practice should be done gently and without force. It is best to practice either early or late in the day, when the air is cool, to keep pitta from overheating. Avoid this exercise if you are experiencing extreme cold or hypothermia. Follow these instructions:

1. Sit comfortably with a long spine.
2. Purse your lips, stick your tongue out, and curl it lengthwise into the shape of a straw.
3. Inhale slowly through the straw and fill your lungs completely.
4. Relax your tongue and draw it back into your mouth, seal your lips, and exhale through your nose very slowly.
5. Repeat this cycle, inhaling though your curled tongue, closing your mouth, and exhaling through your nostrils, for three to five minutes.

If you can't curl your tongue, just keep it relaxed in your mouth and inhale through pursed lips.

Lion's Breath (Simhasana) for Kapha Balance

Lion's Breath prevents kapha accumulation in the body by stimulating the nerves, senses, and mind. It energizes the immune system, which can get sluggish for kapha types. It also relieves tension in the chest and strengthens the lungs, which are the home of kapha in the body. Avoid this breath if you have a recent or chronic injury to the knees, face, neck, or tongue. Follow these instructions:

1. Sit in a comfortable position, either in a chair or kneeling on the floor with your hips on your heels. Ground your weight down into both sitting bones and reach the crown of the head up to lengthen the spine. Take a moment to relax your body.
2. Close your mouth and notice your breath flowing in and out of your nostrils. Allow it to become steady and rhythmic.
3. Place your hands on your thighs with your fingers fanned out.
4. Inhale deeply through your nose as you draw your belly inward and press your chest forward, arching your upper back. Lift your chin, open your eyes wide, and gaze upward at the spot between the eyebrows.
5. Open your mouth and stick out your tongue. Stretch the tip of your tongue down toward the chin, contract the epiglottis in the front of your throat (the swallowing muscles), and slowly exhale all of the breath out, while whispering a loud, strong "Haaaa" sound.
6. Repeat steps 4 and 5 four to six times. Then pause and relax. Close your eyes and let go as you feel the energy flowing through your head, eyes, throat, and belly.

Skull-Shining Breath (Kapalabhati) for Kapha Balance

This is an energizing breath that cleanses the lungs and entire respiratory tract. Skull-Shining Breath improves digestion and metabolism, strengthens the abdominal muscles, and energizes the mind.

Because this is such a powerful pranayama, there are several contraindications. Do not practice this technique if you have any of the following conditions: pregnancy; heart conditions, including hypertension; respiratory conditions; nervous system conditions; recent surgery; inflammation in the abdominal or thoracic regions; or menstruation (the first few days).

Skull-Shining Breath is done by quickly and gently contracting the abdominal muscles during your exhalation and completely relaxing them during your inhalation. This results in a rhythmic pumping of the belly by alternating short, explosive exhalations (expulsions) with slightly longer, and passive, inhalations. The expulsions force the air out of the lungs—creating a vacuum. The release of the abdominal muscles allows for an automatic inhalation to occur as the air sucks back into the lungs to fill the vacuum. Follow these instructions:

1. Sit in a comfortable position with your spine erect. Take a moment to relax your body and tune in to your breath.
2. Seal your lips, and notice your breath flowing in and out of your nostrils. Allow your breath to become steady and deep. You will be breathing through the nostrils throughout this practice.

3. Place one hand on your lower belly to help focus your attention on isolating and contracting this area.

4. Quickly contract your abdominal muscles, pushing a burst of air out of your lungs. Then release the contraction so the belly relaxes, and allow air to passively suck back into your lungs.

5. As you repeat this, let your pace be slow and steady. Repeat fifteen times, creating a comfortable and smooth rhythm. With practice you will become more adept at contracting and releasing your belly.

6. Do one round of fifteen to thirty expulsions to start. Gradually increase to three rounds of thirty expulsions. Allow yourself to take several natural breaths in between each round to integrate the energy of the pranayama.

Three-Part Breath (Dirgha) for All Doshas

Three-Part Breath is good for all doshas, and when done with a focus on long, relaxed exhalations it is especially good for calming the mind and nervous system. Avoid this exercise if you have had recent surgery or injury in your torso or head. Follow these instructions:

1. Sit comfortably with a long spine.
2. Seal your lips and relax your forehead, jaw, and belly.
3. Begin to take steady, long breaths in and out through your nostrils.
4. Let your breath slow down so much that you can feel your belly, rib cage, then chest expand and contract with each inhalation and exhalation.
5. Take a few minutes to establish a relaxed and even breathing rhythm.
6. Next, begin to slow down and extend your exhalations, allowing them to become longer than your inhalations. To help lengthen your exhalations, gently contract your abdominal muscles as you breathe out.
7. Without straining, draw your navel back to the spine to create slow-motion exhalations.
8. Gradually build your exhalations to last twice as long as your inhalations. Stay relaxed as you gently contract your abdominal muscles to squeeze the air out of your lungs. Breathing this way helps to release strong emotions such anger, frustration, and impatience.
9. Continue for three to five minutes.

5

Food and Nutrition

Remember Why You Eat
in the First Place

Can you imagine how you'd feel if you allowed yourself to sit down for every meal, focused on the pleasure of eating and enjoying the moment? Imagine what it would feel like if you were to chew slowly and savor the tastes of every bite. What if you were to learn that making time to sit down and enjoy eating, whether alone or in good company, is not a frivolous way of passing time? In fact, how you eat, coupled with what you eat, is a key factor in a healthy lifestyle. The first steps toward remembering your natural connection to food and its vital role in your health are:

- Become intentional about what foods you eat. Choose whole, natural foods, organic and locally grown when possible.
- Bring the joy back into eating and cooking. Take pleasure in noticing that whole foods are rich in color, diverse in texture, and varied in their delicious tastes.
- Believe in the healing and nourishing power of natural, whole foods. They really are what your body, mind, and spirit need to thrive.

Skip the Processed Foods

Perhaps one of the biggest challenges for you will be not to make processed and adulterated foods a routine part of your diet. If you can shift from eating processed foods to natural and whole foods, you won't have to worry about looking at labels and trying to decipher which meals are good for you and how much surreptitiously added sugar is in each bite. If you have to spend time trying to understand the label, it's a good sign you don't need to be eating that item.

Michael Pollan's *In Defense of Food* is written in a very simple, engaging voice, and he explains very clearly the health benefits of a whole-foods diet. He also explains why our culture has become fixated on calories and ingredients rather than on the benefits of just enjoying and eating real food. The truth is, if you spend your time in the produce section, the bulk foods section (for foods like lentils, nuts, and seeds), and reveling in the seasonal varieties of all-natural whole foods, there isn't any "nutritional value" you have to be worrying about or trying to understand. You can believe in whole foods; they are crafted from nature and have in them what you need.

Ayurveda explains how to best choose foods for you, based on the qualities you find in nature and in yourself.

Slow Down and Savor
the Moment

If you enjoy and appreciate what you're eating while you're eating it, you enhance your body's ability to digest and absorb what your body needs. Create a safe, loving, happy, and relaxed atmosphere at mealtimes.

With a very busy lifestyle, it may be difficult to be in a relaxed mindset when you eat. You may feel you must keep working while you eat, or you may keep walking around the kitchen when you eat. If this is true for you, start by just slowing it down a little bit, sitting down, and taking some deep breaths before you take a bite. This really might not be easy for you. You might think, "Oh, well, that can't be so important, it's just important to know what to eat." Not so. How you eat is important for digestion, elimination, and absorption.

See if you can make this change: Slow down and sit down to focus on eating. It might take some real willpower, and it might mean you mark it in your day planner. Do this for a few days, consistently, at least for two meals a day, and notice what difference occurs for you around eating and in your life. Ahead of time, decide which two meals you will spend a half hour sitting down for and relaxing. Really decide, ahead of time, that this is important. Make that commitment to yourself.

It doesn't have to be a chore to learn how to make good choices: It can be fun and nurturing. Think of it as a way for you to experience more joy in life, every single time you eat, by savoring the effects that food has on your senses of sight, smell, touch, and taste. You really deserve to enjoy your meals, and when you slow down and eat in a way that works for your constitution, you will be able to use food as one of the ways to balance your mood and your energy.

Eat in Moderation

This isn't news, right? Eating in moderation just makes sense. Ayurveda recommends that you eat slowly, chew your food well, and enjoy the tastes. If you slow down and savor what you're eating, it will help you eat less food: You will feel the satisfaction of the smells and tastes, and you won't be shoveling it in mindlessly mouthful after mouthful. Oftentimes if you don't pay attention while you're eating, you could even forget if you have eaten, or soon after you've eaten you may still think you're hungry because you weren't paying attention when you ate. It will help you eat in moderation if you take your time and allow yourself to enjoy the food. Choosing the right foods for your constitution will also help you feel satisfied with appropriate amounts; the tastes and qualities will balance your hunger.

How Much to Eat

A good rule of thumb is to eat about two handfuls of food per meal. To imagine how full your stomach should be after a meal, imagine it as one-third filled with food, one-third filled with warm water, and one-third empty. During your meal, sip warm (or room temperature) water.

Overeating

If you overeat, your stomach will expand, and then it will feel empty even with the appropriate amount of food inside. That will cause you to eat more, and then your stomach will expand more, and so goes the pattern. Eating the right amount is important because you want to give yourself enough of the fuel you need, while being careful not to overload your system with more food than it can digest at a time.

If you notice you don't feel full with two handfuls of food as your guideline, try sipping lemon water throughout the day. Or, if there's a time of day you tend to want to snack, prepare a cup of tea around that time before the hunger strikes. Tulsi tea is a great pick-me-up, and can be a mood enhancer and stress reliever. There are many varieties of tulsi tea available, and some are mixed with other teas for a different kind of flavor and effect. If you want a decaffeinated tea, make sure your tulsi tea is not blended with a caffeinated tea.

MANAGING HIGH VATA ENERGY

If you have high vata energy, you may notice your appetite is variable. When you aren't hungry for breakfast or dinner, drink a cup of warm milk with a teaspoon of cardamom. This soothing and grounding drink will help balance the cool and dry qualities of vata, and give you some nourishment so you won't feel starved later.

Consider Tastes When
You Plan Your Dishes

An important and unique aspect of Ayurveda is the role that tastes play in determining what foods to eat. Ayurveda describes six possible tastes that you can experience (sweet, sour, salty, pungent, bitter, and astringent). Each taste is described in terms of the same elements and qualities of the doshas and the natural elements (such as heating, cooling, dry). Each taste, because of its qualities, will help balance different doshas and affect the digestive fire differently. As always, remember that like increases like and opposites balance. So you'll want to choose tastes with qualities that balance (are opposite to) the elemental qualities of your constitution and elements outside. Of course, be in consultation with your Ayurvedic specialist, because she will also take into consideration what she learns about your digestion and what else is going on in your body, mind, and life. That way she can recommend supportive ways to use the tastes in your diet.

The following information about the tastes provides general guidelines to help you understand the value of tastes and their qualities. Remember, you are unique, and your needs shift with time, seasons, and changes in your life. Talk with your Ayurvedic specialist for more guidance in understanding how the elements are showing up in you, and which tastes would be great for you to favor and which to avoid. The following is a table that shows the six tastes and their associated elements.

Taste	Elements
Sweet	earth and water
Sour	earth and fire
Salty	fire and water
Pungent	air and fire
Bitter	air and ether
Astringent	air and earth

Each taste has more than one effect on the body and mind. Rasa is the actual taste. Virya is the potency in regard to its energy of warming or cooling to the system. Tastes that are more predominant in sweet, bitter, and astringent have a cooling effect. Tastes that are predominant in pungent, salty, and sour have a heating effect.

Vipaka is the post-digestive effect, which may show a different quality than either the rasa or virya and is often very important. The post-digestive effect will become how the foods affect your tissues. There are three types: sweet, sour, pungent. These effects are consistent with how each taste affects you.

- Sweet vipaka comes from sweet and salty tastes.
- Sour vipaka come from sour tastes.
- Pungent vipaka comes from pungent, astringent, and bitter tastes.

Once you become accustomed to the concept of tastes in this way, you will begin to think of food in a whole new light. Soon, you will naturally think of the tastes according to their qualities, just as you begin to see yourself and the world around you in terms of qualities. In this way, you'll see how everything in life is connected.

Examples of Foods and Their Tastes

Ayurveda has observed and documented the qualities of the tastes, and the categorizations are to help choose what's best for you. Because such a treatment of taste is not usually considered in the Western view of a healthy diet, you may not be used to recognizing the tastes in the foods you eat.

Taste	Foods
Sweet	sugar, rice, milk
Sour	lemon, vinegar, pickles
Salty	salt, seaweed, salted snacks (nuts, popcorn)
Pungent	onions, garlic, hot pepper, ginger
Bitter	green, leafy vegetables; neem; aloe vera; black or green tea
Astringent	chickpeas, lentils, peels of fruit, turmeric, cranberries

Each taste, because of its qualities, has a different effect on your body and mind. The easiest way to remember the effects is to think in terms of qualities. If you are running hot, choose tastes that are cooling. If you're feeling sluggish and lethargic, choose tastes that are associated with fire, to add some kick and to stimulate energy in your system.

Tastes for Vata

Remember the qualities associated with vata are cold, dry, light, and mobile. So, you want to ground vata's energy, and balance it with these qualities: warm, moist, and heavy. The tastes that are best for vata are sweet, salty, and sour.

- **Sweet to Ground Vata:** Sweet taste is made up of the elements earth and water, and the sweet taste has moist and heavy qualities both short-term and long-term. These qualities are wonderful for balancing vata's light, mobile, and dry qualities. Sweet has a slightly cooling effect on the digestive system, but just enough to give you a sense of feeling full or satisfied.
- **Sour's Warming and Heavy Support:** Sour's elements are earth and fire, which means sour is grounding and heating, with some moisture. The heating quality of sour helps kindle the digestive fire, making this taste very supportive for vata. The warming and grounding effects stay with the body beyond the process of digestion, also very balancing for vata.

- **Salty Benefits for Vata:** The salty taste is comprised of fire and water. Its initial effects on the system are heating and moistening, which help to balance vata's cool and dry qualities. The fiery element of the salty taste supports digestion, which is very supportive for vata types whose appetites can be variable and whose coolness and dryness affects the digestive fire.

Long-term, the salty taste has a sweet vipaka, which means its post-digestive effects are of those elements of the sweet taste—earth and water. Therefore, long-term, the effects are moistening and grounding (excellent for vata).

These qualities affect the mind, not just the body. So, for example, the grounding quality of sour will create feelings of steadiness and support counteracting vata's tendency toward anxiety and fear.

Which Tastes Are Less Favorable for Vata?

Certain tastes are less favorable than others for vata. You don't have to avoid these tastes altogether, just be mindful about how often you choose these tastes if you're working with vata imbalance:

- **A Little Pungent Is Okay for Vata:** The elements that make up the taste pungent are air and fire, and pungent's vipaka is also pungent. So, the light and airy qualities will be its short- and longer-term effect. Vata doesn't need more air or lightness to stay in the body, so that's why this taste is not highly recommended for vata. Because fire is also an element of pungent, some pungency is all right for vata. Vata could use the heat. To make pungency work for vata, be sure to eat other foods or tastes that are grounding and moistening (to balance the air element).
- **Bitter Is of the Same Elements As Vata:** Bitter is made of the elements of ether and air, and for this reason it's not recommended for vata types. Its vipaka is cooling, so some bitter taste will be fine; you just need to balance it. For example, kale has a bitter taste. So, to make this green food supportive to vata, cook the kale so that it's very warm and moist, oil it well using ghee, and toss in some salt and pumpkin seeds.
- **Astringent Is Too Drying for Vata:** Astringent's elements are earth and air, and its light and drying effects are both short- and long-term because

air is an element that is part of its virya and vipaka. Its vipaka is cooling. Over time it's very drying. Astringent tastes are not thought of as supportive to digestion, and vata needs digestive support. With all the wonderful whole and natural foods available to support vata, it's best to limit your use of astringent tastes when cooking for those with a predominance of vata.

> **WHERE DOES HONEY FALL?**
> Occasionally, there are foods that are exceptions to the rules. In Ayurveda these exceptions are called *prabhav*. Honey falls under this category. Because of its sweet taste, you would expect honey to have a cooling virya. However, honey's virya is heating.

Tastes for Pitta

Remember that pitta's elements are fire and water. Keep in mind that the qualities of the elements that make up pitta include hot, oily, light, mobile, and liquid. When choosing tastes to incorporate into your meal, you'll want to balance these qualities with their opposites.

- **Sweet for Pitta:** Sweet's elements are earth and water. Its virya is cooling, which is a great balance for pitta. Pitta types tend to have a strong appetite and digestion, so the cooling aspect of sweet can help soothe and calm the hunger a little bit. The cooling quality also can help pitta stay balanced and not slide into judgmentalism, anger, and jealousy. As a rule, sweet's vipaka is also sweet, which means it has long-term grounding, moistening, and slightly cooling effects—very good for balancing pitta's mobile, light, and hot qualities.
- **Bitter Cools Down Pitta:** Bitter is a great taste for cooling pitta. Bitter's elements are air and ether, which makes it the coolest of the tastes. Its virya is cooling, and even though its vipaka is pungent, it is recommended to help balance pitta. In small amounts, the bitter taste clears and opens the mind, helping you to see things just as they are. When you begin to see situations in your life for all they offer, the easeful parts and the difficult parts, you can make choices from a better place than you can if you're not seeing so clearly.

- **Astringent Pacifies Pitta:** Astrigent's elements are air and earth. These combine to have a cooling virya, which is wonderful for pitta. Its vipaka is pungent, which means that the airy quality continues and the light and dry qualities have a nice effect for pitta.

Tastes That Aggravate Pitta

Because pitta is of earth and fire, when cooking for predominantly pitta types (and on hot days) choose tastes that aren't heating. The following tastes are not the best to use when cooking for pitta:

- **Sour Creates Heat:** Sour's elements are earth and fire. Its virya and vipaka are heating, which means that it heats up during digestion and continues to have heating qualities after digestion. This isn't what pitta needs. Too much heat for pitta will aggravate the body as well as the mind, potentially leading you to feel jealous, judgmental, angry, and irritated. If you do have sour in your meal, balance it with tastes that can help counteract the heating effects.
- **Salty Is Heating, Then Mild:** Salt's elements are fire and water. With its heating virya, it can be aggravating to pitta. Salt's vipaka is sweet, which means it cools down after digestion. Sweet is a grounding taste that is good for pitta's diet, so some salty taste in moderation would be fine for pitta. Every person is different, though, so take note of how it affects you.
- **No Pungent for Pitta:** Of all the tastes, pungent is the hottest, with elements of air and fire. You don't want to make a pungent dish in the middle of summertime for lunch if you're already experiencing a predominance of pitta in your constitution. If you serve pungent dishes to someone who is predominantly pitta, you really want to balance it with other tastes or foods. The taste pungent has a vipaka that is pungent: The qualities it engenders even after digestion are heating, light, and dry.

Tastes for Kapha

Kapha's elements are water and earth. Kapha is stable, damp, and cold. When choosing tastes for kapha, the best tastes are those that will have heating and slightly drying qualities. These balance the heavy and moist kapha qualities.

- **Pungent to Heat Kapha:** Pungent, as the hottest of the tastes, is a great match for a kapha type. It will help with digestion and an overall heating of the body. Pungent's elements are air and fire, which makes it hot, dry, and mobile. Pungent's vipaka is still pungent, so the heating and drying effects are powerful and long-lasting. That's good news for kapha!
- **You Can Lighten Up with Bitter:** Bitter taste has light and dry qualities, so it's a good taste for kapha types. Its elements are air and ether, which means it also has the quality of coolness. Even though kapha is already cool, bitter taste is very supportive because it's drying and light from beginning to end—balancing the water and earth elements of kapha. Its vipaka is pungent, so the long-term qualities are very supportive to kapha: light, dry, heating.
- **Astringent Works for Kapha:** Astringent and kapha both are made up of earth as one of their two elements. Astringent is a good balance for kapha because astringent's other element is air. Kapha's is water. The air element creates lightness and dryness, a great balance for kapha's water element. Like bitter, astringent has a pungent vipaka. So at first astringent will have a cooling effect on the body and on digestion, and then its post-digestive qualities are heating, dry, and light. That's the opposite, and thus a good support, to kapha.

KIDS AND KAPHA

Since childhood is the kapha time of life, pungent is a taste to think about adding when you are preparing children's meals. Adding the pungent taste can be done as easily as flavoring dishes with garlic and onions.

Tastes That Don't Support Kapha

Kapha is made of the stable element earth and the lubricating element water. If you are feeling the effects of the kapha dosha, you don't want to choose tastes that are going to increase the heavy and liquid qualities. This can cause depression, lethargy, weight gain, and possessiveness. So, be mindful of the following tastes in your diet. If you choose them, then be sure to also have some lighter, drying, and heating tastes/foods as well.

- **Kapha Doesn't Need Sweetness:** A kapha individual can be a very grounded and nurturing personality. He doesn't need more sweetness; he already has a wonderful amount. Sweet's elements are the same as kapha's: earth and water as its virya and vipaka. These two elements together help a body bulk up with weight gain, when eaten in excess, and can lead to inertia. A little bit of sweet is fine, at the end of a meal, to help you feel satisfied, but it's best that your meals not include a lot of this taste.
- **Sour and Kapha:** Sour has a warming effect on the body, which could be a nice balance to kapha. However, sour in general has a heavy, grounded, and moist feel to it. Its elements are earth and fire. And the grounded and unctuous qualities of sour could be too much for kapha. If you do want to include sour in your meal—for you, your kapha friend, or a child—it would be best to find a way to balance it using other tastes or foods.
- **Salty Taste Shares Kapha's Heaviness:** One of the effects of the salty taste is that it helps the body retain water. Kapha, being of earth and water, does not need help retaining water. Extra salt in the kapha diet will create more of what kapha already has. Though the elements of salt's intial taste are fire and water, which means the fire will initially feel heating for kapha, salt's vipaka is sweet: very heavy and moist. That means, post-digestion, salt's qualities are earth and water—increasing what kapha already has naturally, taking it to excess.

Stock Your Kitchen Wisely

If Ayurvedic cooking is new to you, you may not have the usual go-to ingredients in your kitchen. Once you have the basics on hand, however, you'll have all you need at your fingertips to make meals that will be delicious and balancing for all types. Specific spices, herbs, and oils are key ingredients to keep in the cupboard so you can tailor meals. You will use the staples both in everyday meals and as support if you are noticing imbalance, e.g., if you catch a cold, have mild digestive issues, or can't fall asleep.

Spices and Herbs

The wisdom of Ayurveda explains how to use spices and herbs both as delicious components of a meal and as a necessary means to health and longevity. Following are the typical herbs and spices you will reach for again and again.

- ○ Basil
- ○ Black pepper
- ○ Cardamom
- ○ Cinnamon
- ○ Clove
- ○ Coriander
- ○ Cumin
- ○ Fennel
- ○ Ginger
- ○ Mint leaves
- ○ Nutmeg
- ○ Raw sugar
- ○ Sea salt
- ○ Thyme
- ○ Turmeric

BUYING, GRINDING, AND MIXING SPICES

If you buy your spices whole, you can use a mortar and pestle to grind them and mix them with other spices. When you grind the spices this way, as you use your own muscle power, be consciously aware of putting healing and loving energy into the spices with every stroke. Another option for grinding whole spices is to use an electric spice grinder.

Depending on which doshas you are working to balance, and depending on what your tastes are, some of these spices you may favor more than others. You also may favor some more than others depending on the season.

Most of the spices and herbs that you'll need are available in grocery stores near you. Dry spices will typically be in the spice aisle, in glass jars. If you buy spices fresh, they may be in a refrigerated section. You can also buy spices online. Some sites to search are:

- Banyan Botanicals: www.banyanbotanicals.com
- Penzeys: www.penzeys.com
- Dean & Deluca: www.deandeluca.com
- The Spice House: www.thespicehouse.com

Buy the freshest and highest quality spices that you can afford.

HOW TO STORE SPICES

Store your spices in airtight glass or plastic containers. Keep them in a cool place: in a drawer or cabinet (out of the sunlight). Also, label the contents of each container clearly, and put the date on the label too. Your spices will stay fresh enough for about six months to one year.

Dry Legumes to Keep Stocked

Legumes are one of the main ways you'll be getting your protein. Before you cook legumes, be sure to rinse them and pick out any debris. It will be easier to cook and digest some legumes if you soak them first for a few hours. Here are some staple legumes for you to have available:

- Red, brown, or black lentils
- Mung dahl
- Adzuki beans
- Black beans
- Split peas
- Chickpeas

Legumes are such a good part of any meal because you can doctor them up with spices, mix them with rice, and/or add vegetables to them. You can prepare them like a stew on cold nights, or make lighter recipes other times of the year and use them as side dishes or appetizers (e.g., hummus or bean dip).

Grains

Grains provide you with a variety of nutrients and can be seasoned to be either sweet or savory, depending on your tastes and your body's needs. Amaranth, millet, and quinoa, for example, are gluten-free and provide you with a good dose of protein to boot! In addition to important vitamins, minerals, and healthy fats, whole grains provide a good dose of fiber. Some high-fiber grains are: amaranth, brown rice, buckwheat, millet, quinoa, spelt, whole rye, steel-cut oats and rolled oats (even instant oatmeal), and whole-wheat couscous.

Whole grains are incredibly versatile. You can eat them as breakfast cereal, as part of a lunch burrito or midday salad, or mixed together with vegetables or legumes for dinner. Here is a list of grains to have in your cupboard:

- Amaranth
- Millet
- Whole oats
- Quinoa
- Basmati rice
- Brown rice

If some of these grains are new to you and you don't like the first recipe you try, keep in mind that you may like the grain in a different recipe.

Nuts and Seeds

Nuts and seeds are wonderful to be used as a snack or as a part of your meal. Which nuts and seeds you choose will depend on your constitution.

Dosha	Nuts	Seeds
Vata	almonds, black walnuts, Brazil nuts, cashews, charole, coconut, filberts, hazelnuts, macadamia nuts, peanuts, pecans, pine nuts, pistachios, walnuts	chia, flax, halva, pumpkin, sesame, sunflower, tahini
Pitta	almonds (soaked and peeled), charole, coconut	flax, halva, popcorn (buttered, no salt), psyllium, pumpkin, sunflower
Kapha	charole	chia, flax, popcorn (buttered, no salt), pumpkin, sunflower

Taken from *The Complete Book of Ayurvedic Home Remedies* by Dr. Vasant Lad

Ghee and Oils

Ghee and oils are very nourishing, supportive, and balancing. Keep the oils stocked that are most needed for you and your family, based on constitution.

HOW TO MAKE GHEE

1. Put 1 pound sweet, unsalted butter into a medium-sized pot. On medium heat, melt the butter, without burning it.
2. Allow the butter to boil. Stir occasionally, as the butter boils and sputters a bit.
3. Soon you'll notice the ghee becoming a clear golden color and white solid pieces will form. When the bubbling has quieted down, the ghee is ready. This whole process takes about 10–15 minutes.
4. Remove the ghee from the heat immediately. At this stage it's prone to burn. Let the ghee cool slightly.
5. Pour the ghee through cheesecloth or a metal strainer into a clean, glass jar, separating the solids from the clear ghee.
6. Store at room temperature, and when you spoon ghee out, make sure the spoon is clean and dry.

- **Oils for Vata:** Vata does well with a lot of oil. To combat the dry and cool qualities, keep sesame oil stocked for self-massage. At meals, vatas can put a healthy helping of ghee in their food. Use it to sauté or cook with instead of butter, and drop a half a tablespoon into your dish when the food is piping hot and ready to eat. Ghee can be used in most anything from grains to vegetables to legumes. Olive oil and sesame oil are the two oils to favor when cooking for vata. Most oils will work well for vata; however, avoid coconut oil when preparing food for vata.
- **Oils for Pitta:** Pitta does well with most oils. As is the case with vata, ghee can be used often for pitta. Sunflower oil is the best for pitta. Canola, olive, flaxseed, and walnut oils are also good to cook with for pitta. The best oils for pitta's self-massage are sunflower and coconut.

- **Oils for Kapha:** Kapha doesn't need a lot of extra oil. A bit of oil will be good for kapha, even though kapha is already moist. Corn, canola, and sesame are the best oils for kapha. Ghee won't harm kapha—ghee is good for all doshas. Olive oil is not a good balancing oil for kapha.

Vegetables, Fruits, and Berries

Get organic, locally grown whole vegetables, fruits, and berries when possible. Buy what is in season, and choose an assortment of foods that naturally come in a variety of colors. Keep in mind, of course, your constitution and the constitution of those for whom you are cooking. If you don't cook at home every night, buy frozen vegetables, fruits, and berries because they will last longer. Read the packages to get what is most fresh, whole, and natural.

Nut and Seed Butters

Nut butters are versatile. They are perfect on vegetables and fruit. Peanut butter isn't the only nut or seed butter available, though it's very popular in the West. Almond and sunflower butters are also delicious and great options. Choose which nut is best for your constitution, and keep nut butter in the refrigerator once opened.

Natural Sweeteners

Sweet is a great taste for vata and pitta types. Kapha would do well to go lightly with sweets, but all doshas can use all of the six tastes. So, having sweeteners around is good for everyone.

Dosha	Sweetener
Vata	honey, molasses, rice syrup
Pitta	maple syrup, rice syrup
Kapha	honey

Remember that sweet is also one of the six tastes, so you can find sweet in foods without adding sweetener when you're craving the sweet taste.

Customize Meals with Spice Mixes

Masala is a term used to describe a spice blend or spice mixture. You can use spice mixtures to enhance the flavor of food, to improve digestion, and for their therapeutic properties (such as carminative, alterative, diuretic, or analgesic). Using the right spices in your diet will help you maintain strong digestive fire, reduce toxins, and bring balance to the doshas.

How to Cook with Masalas

One of the best ways to cook with masalas is to sauté the blends in some ghee (clarified butter) or oil. The ghee or oil helps to extract the flavors and aromas of these spices while releasing the natural oils, which contain many of the therapeutic components. Once you mix the spices in ghee or oil, add vegetables or your choice of other food to the mixture and sauté. Masalas can also be added to soups, stews, rice, or kitchari.

You can customize spice blends so they will help pacify any doshic imbalance, or vikruti, to suit your taste. For example, a person who is experiencing high kapha may want to use a kapha-reducing masala. Here are masala recipes for each dosha.

MASALA FOR VATA TYPE
- 2 tablespoons cumin
- 1 tablespoon turmeric
- 1 tablespoon fennel
- 1 teaspoon asafoetida
- 1 teaspoon ginger
- 1 teaspoon sesame seeds
- ½ teaspoon mineral salt

MASALA FOR PITTA TYPE

- 2 tablespoons coriander
- 1 tablespoon cumin
- 1 tablespoon turmeric
- 1 tablespoon fennel
- 1 teaspoon cardamom
- 1 teaspoon raw sugar
- ¼ teaspoon clove

MASALA FOR KAPHA TYPE

- 1 tablespoon turmeric
- 1 tablespoon coriander
- 1 tablespoon fennel
- 1 teaspoon cinnamon
- 1 teaspoon cumin
- 1 teaspoon ginger

To save time, make several servings of these masalas ahead of time, and keep them for up to six months. Have them nearby with your other spices, so you can easily reach for them when you're cooking. Here are more tips when making spice masalas:

- It's best to use the powdered form of the spices. If you can, buy whole spices in bulk and grind them using a spice grinder or a mortar and pestle.
- Organic and nonirradiated spices are of the best quality.
- Store masalas in a sealed container in a cool, dark place.

Spice blends are delicious, nutritious, and fun to use. Because they have an array of therapeutic benefits for the body, mind, and senses, it's no wonder that spices in times of trade have been valued as highly as gold.

❋

Make Your Own
Teas and Brews

Drinking tea or brews is an important part of your Ayurvedic lifestyle. By drinking teas and brews, you can bring balance to your doshas, energize yourself during the day, and relax yourself before going to bed. There are so many recipes for brews and teas that Ayurveda suggests, and having some ingredients on hand can be helpful for when you need just the right warm drink. Choose organic as often as possible.

Store-Bought Teas

The grocery store has a variety of teas available. Good choices to have on hand are peppermint tea (can ease digestive discomfort and help you relax at bedtime), ginger tea (to support digestion), and tulsi tea (also called "holy basil," used for a variety of health benefits, including helping to give you a boost if you are low on energy). Following are some companies to support your quest:

- The brand Traditional Medicinals has a variety of teas made to help support your health: www.traditionalmedicinals.com
- The Chopra Center has organic teas for balancing each dosha: https://store.chopra.com
- Pukka is a UK brand named for its commitment to "authentic" and "genuine" practice and products: www.pukkaherbs.com
- Rishi Tea sells organic fair trade teas: www.rishi-tea.com
- Harney & Sons has paired up with the Chopra Center, creating Ayurvedic-inspired blends, and they have a large assortment of other teas as well: www.harney.com

DIY Blends

You also have the option of making your own blends, simply and with love. To make your own tea you'll need a teapot, and either a strainer, a tea infuser, or tea filters (you can buy one made of reusable cloth or those made of biodegradable paper). Some teapots come with their own strainer or infuser. To use those, put your herbs into the strainer, pour boiling water over it, and let it steep for the desired amount of time. Then, when you pour the tea into your mug, the herbs stay in the strainer. If you don't want to use a strainer, you can buy reusable or biodegradable tea bags to put your herbs in for individual cups of tea.

You can make your own simple brews by putting your desired herbs in boiling water or warm milk and letting them steep. As you prepare for bed, make yourself mint tea by putting mint in the tea filter or infuser, pouring boiling water over it, then letting it steep for five to seven minutes before drinking. Here are two teas that can help all doshas:

- Make your own **ginger brew** by grating 2 teaspoons of fresh ginger, putting it in the bottom of a mug, then pouring boiling water over it and letting it steep for 10 minutes. To add some complexity to the brew, after 10 minutes, add 2 teaspoons of honey and a few squirts of lemon juice. (You could also drink the ginger brew without the honey and lemon.) A great time to drink this brew would be a half hour before a meal, to get the digestive fire stimulated.
- **Cumin, coriander, fennel tea** is a common brew to take for helping digestion. You can take this once per day (or as recommended by your specialist) to help remove toxins from the body in a very gentle way. To make this tea, put 1 teaspoon each of cumin, coriander, and fennel into your strainer or filter, then steep in boiling water for about 10 to 15 minutes. A good time to drink this brew is about a half hour after finishing your meal.

Some herbs are stronger than others, so it's best to talk with your Ayurvedic specialist before experimenting. She can tell you which herbs to take in tea on a regular basis, and which to be more cautious about, especially when considering your constitution.

De-Stress with Ashwagandha

Ashwagandha (*Withania somnifera*) is a soothing adaptogen (a natural substance that helps the body manage stress—a common example is ginseng). Nervous system challenges such as anxiety, fatigue, and insomnia from stress are all reasons an Ayurvedic specialist might suggest ashwagandha. Here are other uses:

- Enhancing endocrine function
- Supporting an underactive thyroid and balanced functioning for the testes and adrenal glands
- Offering fertility and vitality in men
- Providing iron during heavy menstrual periods
- Giving immune support for either hyper- or hypo-immune function

Ashwagandha can be grown as an annual in cooler climates.

SAFETY NOTE

As with all herbs, it's important to talk with a certified expert before adding ashwaganda into your diet or administering it to your family. Ashwaganda is part of the nightshade family alongside tomatoes, peppers, and potatoes, so if you have allergies to plants in this family you may want to consider other options. Ashwagandha can stimulate the thyroid gland and it's very high in iron, so consult with your doctor or Ayurvedic specialist before taking it. And although sometimes used as a fertility tonic, this herb may not be suitable for use during pregnancy.

Ashwagandha is so popular that it can be found in different forms, such as extracts, powders, capsules, and teas, and it is often mixed with other herbs to complement their properties and ameliorate a variety of symptoms.

6

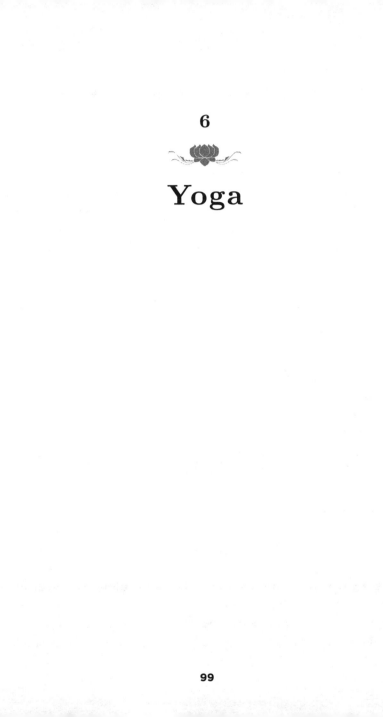

Yoga

Enjoy Stillness with Yoga

The images of yogis twisting and bending their bodies into various shapes may lead you to imagine that yoga is a practice exclusively for the body. It's true that the physical postures of yoga are intended to release toxins from the body, create space, and lead to other physical benefits. It's also true that hatha yoga, the physical practice of yoga, illuminates the nature of the mind.

To understand the mind, you have to practice observing it. As you practice hatha yoga, you are able to watch your mind and watch what thoughts arise as you flow from posture to posture. Can you keep your mind steady and present, or does it wander and become restless? Can you return your attention to the breath, and become present simply to the experience, without judging it? During your hatha yoga practice, observe that the mind likes to travel.

STAY IN THE PRESENT

During your hatha yoga practice, when your mind wanders, bring it back to the moment by noticing what parts of your body are touching the earth. Feel the support of the earth, then follow the breath. In hatha yoga, your breath supports your postures. You'll learn to coordinate your movements with your inhalation and exhalation for safety, ease, and stamina.

Hatha yoga also is a practice to prepare the body for stillness. By first moving the body in hatha yoga, you will have an easier time sitting in stillness. From stillness, you observe the nature of the mind. You watch thoughts go by, without getting attached to them or continuing to follow where they will lead. Every time you notice you have a thought, just bring your awareness back to your breath. Notice you are breathing, and watch the inhalation and exhalation. Notice the pause at the end of the inhalation and the end of the exhalation. As thoughts arise, gently bring your attention back to the breath.

The mind is restless. It plans. It thinks. It worries. There's a time and place for those functions of the mind. It's wonderful that the mind can be so adept and supportive of work and productivity. It's also important for you to learn how to create conditions so that the mind will rest, especially if it starts to spin in a stressful situation. Once you understand the nature of the mind, you are on your way to understanding how yoga and meditation are tools for the reduction of stress. Understanding this concept will support your Ayurvedic lifestyle. If you practice both Ayurveda and yoga, they support and enhance each other's effects, taking you toward deeper health of body, mind, and spirit.

How Yoga Reduces Mental Stress

Would you like better coping skills in the face of life's ups and downs? Would you like relief from spirals of depressive thoughts and anxiety? Would you like to know how to let go of anger and resentment? Yoga is here with the tools to help you.

Yoga teaches that in order to reduce the stress you feel, you must understand the nature of the mind. In your life, you will find yourself in situations that could lead you to feel stressed-out, depressed, hopeless, alone, fearful, and anxious. You cannot control all the situations and outcomes in your life. Yoga teaches that you can learn practices designed to help you more effectively manage the stress you feel as a result of what happens beyond your control. When you understand the nature of the mind, you can change your experience of life and experience it with more joy, playfulness, and ease.

What Are the Yoga Sutras?

The *Yoga Sutras* were written by Patanjali in Sanskrit thousands of years ago (estimated dates range from 500 B.C. to A.D. 300), and now there are several translations and editions available in English. The *Yoga Sutras* were written to explain the science and philosophy of yoga. Patanjali didn't invent the study of yoga, but he is credited with writing it down in the poetic form that we have today. Each sutra is as short as one phrase or a few sentences, and they are threads of wisdom for you to contemplate as you move along your yogic journey toward understanding the nature of the mind. Here are the basic premises to understanding the nature of the mind, which is foundational to your peace of mind and your practice of Ayurveda, the science of life:

- You are not your thoughts; you are the one who can observe your thoughts.
- The mind is active—thinking, planning, judging, hoping, fearing, desiring, avoiding.
- When the mind is actively fearful, anxious, stressed, etc., that is not your true nature.
- Your true nature is Purusha, pure awareness.
- In order to experience pure awareness, you must learn to observe and calm the mind.
- Once the mind is calm, you experience peace, not stress, in your life.

Yoga and meditation are tools for learning to develop what is often called "witness consciousness," which is a way of saying that you are the witness to what is going on in your life. You are witnessing your thoughts, your reactions, and your emotions. You are not identifying yourself with them, as though you are them, nor are you getting caught up in them. You begin to recognize that your anger, your resentment, your guilt, your insecurity, etc., are not your natural state of mind. You, at your core, are at peace and equilibrium. Yoga and meditation teach you how to get in touch with that core and live from that place more often.

Warm Up

Always begin your yoga practice with a warm-up. Keep it moderate—nothing too heating or challenging. For example, a great warm-up for pitta types would be to rotate and loosen up all of the joints in the body. Be sure to include your ankles, knees, hips, wrists, elbows, shoulders, neck, and spine.

Once warmed up, become still, soften your gaze on the horizon, and bring your awareness to your breath. Take a few minutes to cultivate a steady and slow breathing rhythm. Once you have established your breath, begin to slow down and lengthen your exhalations by drawing your navel toward the spine as you breathe out. This technique of elongated, slow-motion exhalations should be used throughout the following sequence to help calm your body and nervous system.

Customize Your Practice

Yoga is not "one size fits all," Janna Delgado, yoga and Ayurvedic specialist at Kripalu Center for Yoga & Health, explains, meaning that you can choose particular postures and practices depending on what you need for balance. For example, a vata practice should be steady and grounding to keep you stable; a pitta practice should have an internal focus on surrender and nonjudgment to cool your competitive nature; and a kapha practice should be active and warming to awaken your energy.

Cool Down

- **Vata:** The perfect cooldown for vata is yoga nidra, or yogic sleep. It's a guided practice. As you lie down in Savasana, you are guided to relax the body so much that you enter that special state that is not quite awake and not quite asleep. It is here where deep relaxation and bliss occur. In the absence of having a CD or teacher to guide you in yoga nidra, you can do a body scan. Lie down and put a blanket over your body. Once you are comfortable, envision each body part head to toe, and as you get to each part of the body, take a deep inhale and long exhale and invite relaxation into that space.

- **Pitta:** Pitta types need plenty of time for relaxation and integration at the end of a practice to allow accumulated pitta to completely release. Be sure to rest in Savasana, lying on your back, for at least fifteen minutes with a soft, relaxed breath. Allow yourself to completely let go and surrender into stillness.

- **Kapha:** Mellow Kaphas will be happy to hear that Savasana, or Corpse Pose, is one of the most important postures. It's where the real integration and rebalancing of the doshas takes place. To practice, lie face-up on the floor with your arms and legs extended, and your palms facing up. Allow yourself to release tension and completely relax. Let go of everything, including control of the breath. Imagine your body can breathe itself. Enjoy Corpse Pose for five to fifteen minutes, longer if you have time.

Safety Note

Consult with your doctors and healers before doing yoga. During practice, if you feel any sharp pain, stop what you're doing and relax. Consult your doctor before taking on any new physical practice, like yoga, and especially if you are pregnant or have cardiovascular or respiratory conditions.

Tadasana: Mountain Pose for Vata

Most poses are good for balancing vata. Some are more inherently calming and grounding. As vata "resides" in the large intestine, pelvic area, and lower abdomen, poses that compress or stretch these areas will help balance vata. Poses to be avoided or modified are those that are overly stimulating to the nervous system, such as rapid vinyasa sequences (transitions between different poses) or postures that put excessive pressure on the joints—especially the neck, shoulders, and knees.

1. Stand with your feet hip-width distance apart. Feel your feet, especially the base of the big toe, firmly planted on the ground.
2. Engage the legs, tuck your tailbone under slightly, and lift up through the crown of your head.
3. Inhale and lift the shoulders up.
4. Exhale and roll the shoulders back and down.
5. Inhale. On the exhalation, with your arms by your sides, extend the fingers so that the fingertips point toward the earth. Feel the downward energy grounding you.
6. Take nice, long, deep breaths in and out, as you gently fix your gaze out in front of you.
7. Envision yourself tall, strong, and heavy like a mountain—grounded in the earth and majestically connected to the sky. Keep breathing.
8. After several breaths in Mountain Pose *(see image on page 6 of the insert)*, stay standing and relax the posture. Notice how you feel.

Virabhadrasana I: Warrior I Pose for Vata

As you come into this pose, imagine yourself a warrior: impressively strong and focused. Feel the heat rising as you hold the posture, and feel the earth supporting you.

1. Start standing in Tadasana (Mountain Pose) with your feet hip-width distance apart and firmly pressing into the floor.
2. Place your hands on your hips; inhale. On the exhalation, take a big step back with your left foot; keep both feet pointing forward.
3. Press the base of the big and little toes of the front foot firmly into the floor. The heel of the back foot should press toward the floor. For greater stability, place a rolled towel or small cushion under the back heel. Align your hips so they face directly forward.
4. Keeping a strong abdominal core, lift the arms out to the sides and overhead in a "V" position, palms facing each other *(see image on page 6 of the insert)*.
5. Continue to breathe with a steady inhalation and exhalation. Maintain a soft gaze on one spot.
6. To release this posture, lower the arms to your sides or hips, and on the exhalation step the back foot up to meet the front.
7. Repeat the Warrior I Pose, this time taking a big step back with the right foot.

Child's Pose for Vata

To pacify a vata imbalance, the key is to remember that less is more. Practice surrendering rather than striving, and focus on acceptance rather than judgment.

1. Start on all fours, with the hands under the shoulders and the knees under the hips. Keep your knees on the floor, bent at 90-degree angles, with the hips aligned over the knees. With knees either together or apart, lower your hips onto your heels. (If your sitting bones don't reach your heels, put a small cushion on top of your heels so your sitting bones can rest on that cushion.) Straighten you arms out in front of you, in line with your shoulders.

2. Keep your hands on the floor, arms stretched out over your head, as you place your forehead on the earth *(see image on page 8 of the insert)*. Feel the earth supporting you at all the points where you're touching the ground. (If your forehead doesn't touch the earth, you can prop your forehead up with your hands, or use a cushion here too.)

3. Take some long, deep breaths, so deep it might feel like you are filling the lower back and lungs with air. Take several steady breaths.

4. To release this posture, come up to hands and knees, and then lie down on your right side in the fetal position to rest.

Uttanasana: Standing Wide-Angle Forward Fold for Pitta

Before doing any postures, it's important to know the benefits and the contra-indications. Benefits of Standing Wide-Angle Forward Fold include the following: the pose cools and circulates abdominal energy, it calms an overheated brain, and it sends excess heat down the energy channels in the legs and into the earth. Contraindication for Standing Wide-Angle Forward Fold is that those suffering from lower-back issues should either avoid this pose, or keep the knees bent while practicing it.

1. Stand with your feet 3 to 4 feet apart with hands on your hips.
2. Bring your feet parallel to each other and press the outer edges of your feet firmly into the floor.
3. Firm up your thigh muscles.
4. Inhale and lift your chest.
5. Hinging at the hips, exhale and lift your tailbone as you fold forward, keeping your spine long.
6. When your torso is parallel to the floor, place your hands on the floor directly below your shoulders. (Place your hands on blocks or thick books as a modification. Or, if the backs of your legs or spine are tight, bend your knees.)
7. Distribute your weight evenly between your hands and feet. Work to lengthen your arms and legs.
8. Widen your shoulder blades across your back and draw your shoulders away from your ears.

9. Gaze straight down and lengthen your spine from the tip of your tailbone through the crown of your head *(see image on page 8 of the insert)*.

10. Stay in the pose for five to ten deep breaths, with an emphasis on longer exhalations for a cooling effect.

You can proceed directly to the next posture, Twisting Wide-Angle Forward Fold, or come out and rest first. To come out of the pose, press your feet into the floor and bring your hands to your hips. Inhale and press your tailbone down toward the floor, as you lift your torso up to vertical. Step your feet together, close your eyes, and feel the effects of the pose.

Twisting Wide-Angle Forward Fold for Pitta

Because pitta types have a tendency to overheat by pushing themselves way too hard, they benefit most from a cooling, calming, and relaxed yoga practice. Softer poses help reduce the heat and emotional intensity that pitta types are prone to.

The benefits of twisting are that it massages the organs of digestion, which are where pitta lives in the body. Twists help you avoid overheating or becoming overly aggressive, because they wring out excess heat. The contraindications are for those suffering from issues of the spine and pregnant women: These people should avoid this pose.

1. Come into Standing Wide-Angle Forward Fold, as previously described, with your hands on the floor (or blocks) below your shoulders, your feet firmly planted on the floor, and your torso elongated.

2. Lift your left hand and place it on the floor on the outside of your right hand, pressing your palm firmly down into the floor. If there is tension in your lower back or legs, bend your knees a bit.

3. Exhale and sweep your right hand up toward the ceiling. Revolve your spine and extend up through your arm *(see image on page 8 of the insert)*.

4. Breathe deeply for five to ten breaths, elongating your exhalations to help decompress pitta.

5. Release by lowering your right arm on an inhalation.

6. Return to Standing Wide-Angle Forward Fold Pose for one complete breath.

7. Repeat the above steps, twisting to the other side (your left side) for five to ten breaths, focusing on long exhalations to calm your nervous system.

8. To come out, release your left arm toward the floor and return to Standing Wide-Angle Forward Fold.

9. Place your hands on your hips, inhale, and press your tailbone down toward the floor as you lift the torso up to vertical.

10. Step your feet together. Pause to feel the effects of the forward fold and twist.

Reclined Twist for Pitta

This twist is great for pitta types because it's calming and not overly heating. Twists release excess pitta from the digestive organs, which are the seat of pitta in the body. If you are pregnant or experiencing any hip or back pain, stop practicing and consult a physician.

1. To begin, lie on your back with your knees bent and your feet on the floor. If there is tension in your neck and shoulders, place a folded blanket or thin pillow under your head.
2. Take a few moments to breathe deeply to melt away any tension. Feel the muscles in the back of your body soften and spread out.
3. Draw both knees into your chest.
4. Take your arms out to the sides, on the floor, perpendicular to your body, with palms facing up. Inhale deeply.
5. Exhale slowly as you release your hips and let your knees drop over to the right side.
6. Place your right hand on your left knee, keeping both shoulders flat on the floor (see image on page 8 of the insert).
7. Turn your head to the left if it feels comfortable.
8. Soften and surrender as you breathe quietly here. Without straining, draw your navel toward your spine on each exhalation to create a slow-motion and complete exhalation.
9. Take five to ten breaths, drawing your awareness inward to focus on the sensation of your breath.
10. Return to center on an inhalation and repeat on the other side.

When you've completed both sides, draw both knees to your chest and rock gently from side to side for a few breaths. Then release your arms and legs on the floor and relax for a few breaths.

Sun Salutation for Kapha

Come into standing, with a tall spine and your feet hip-width distance apart. Bring your awareness to your breath. Seal your lips and breathe slowly through your nostrils. Stabilize and smooth out your breath. Once you have established a steady rhythm, begin strengthening your exhalations by slowly drawing your navel back toward your spine as you breathe out. This abdominal contraction on exhalation will help establish inner heat to melt away excess kapha. Unless noted, breathe this way throughout the following warm-up and yoga sequence.

The Sun Salutation is a fantastic way to get kapha types moving and warm themselves up. The twelve postures in the sequence effectively stretch, strengthen, and massage all of the joints, muscles, and internal organs of the body. Other benefits include nourishing and balancing the endocrine, circulatory, respiratory, digestive, and immune systems. Move slowly through the sequence, with a focus on deep and steady breathing, to stoke inner heat.

1. Stand in Mountain Pose *(see image on page 6 of the insert)* with feet hip-width distance apart and parallel. Distribute the weight evenly between the balls and heels of each foot. Engage the legs and lengthen the spine. Stand tall with relaxed shoulders. Bring your palms together in front of the heart. Notice your breath. Begin taking slow, deep breaths. Use this breath to establish a steady rhythm for the sequence.

2. Inhale and raise the arms out to the sides and up overhead. Press down through the feet, lift out of the waist, and lengthen the fingertips to the sky.

3. Exhale and swan dive forward, sweeping the arms out to the sides as you hinge forward from the hips coming into a Standing Forward

Fold *(see image on page 6 of the insert)*. Place your hands on the floor or your shins. If the hamstrings are tight, bend the knees a bit or use blocks as props underneath your hands.

4. Inhale, press down through the hands and feet, look forward, and lengthen the spine, lifting up halfway into a jackknife position.

5. Exhale and return to Standing Forward Fold, gently drawing the torso toward the thighs.

6. Bend the knees and bring the palms to the floor, framing the feet.

7. Inhale and step the left foot back into a lunge. Sweep the arms forward and overhead for Warrior I *(see image on page 6 of the insert)*. The heart lifts while the shoulders and hips sink into gravity. You may wish to place the left knee on the floor to modify the lunge.

8. Exhale, sweep the palms down to the floor to frame the foot, and step the right foot back into Plank Pose *(see image on page 7 of the insert)*, or push-up position. Breathe. To modify, bring the knees to the floor.

9. Exhale and lower to the earth, landing the hips, ribs, and chest all at the same time. Elbows stay close by the sides, fingers spread wide.

10. Plant the palms and pubic bone. Inhale and peel the forehead, chin, and chest away from the earth. Keep the elbows in toward the ribs and the shoulders relaxed.

11. Exhale, curl the toes under, press palms into the ground, and lift the hips toward the sky, coming into Downward Facing Dog *(see image on page 7 of the insert)*. Breathe deeply in this pose. Press the belly and chest back toward the thighs. Lengthen the spine from the crown of the head through the tip of the tailbone. Relax the shoulder blades down the back. Root the palms and heels down.

12. Inhale and step the left foot between the hands for lunge. You may need to reach back and help the foot step all the way forward. Arms sweep forward and overhead for Warrior I. Lift up through the chest and the crown. Let the shoulders and tailbone relax down. To modify the lunge, simply lower the right knee to the floor.

13. Exhale and sweep the hands to the floor, step the right foot beside the left, coming into Standing Forward Fold. Place the hands alongside the feet or on the shins.

14. Inhale and look up as you lift the chest and straighten the arms and legs, coming into jackknife. Root down through the palms and feet. Keep a long spine.

15. Exhale and release back down into Standing Forward Fold. Gently press the belly toward the thighs and the heart toward the shins. Bend the knees slightly if you need to.

16. Ground through the feet and legs. Inhale and sweep the arms out to the sides and overhead as you press all the way up to standing. Palms touch overhead.

17. Exhale and lower the palms down to the heart. Pause.

18. Repeat the sequence once more, leading with the right leg this time. Don't be afraid to break a sweat and challenge yourself!

19. Pause and relax. With your awareness, follow the flow of your breath, letting it gradually slow down. Tune in to the flow of energy throughout your body and mind.

KAPHA YOGA

Janna Delgado, yoga and Ayurvedic specialist at Kripalu Center for Yoga & Health, instructs, "Kaphas should practice in an energetic way, putting in their full effort and pushing beyond their comfort zone." Janna uses the following yoga and breathwork flows to help kaphas focus on coordinating breath with movements to build heat, circulate energy, and fire up metabolism. The flows will also open up the heart, chest, and lungs—all the places where kapha tends to accumulate.

Angel Breaths for Kapha

Angel Breaths stimulate and tone the heart, diaphragm, and abdominal organs—all of the places that kapha likes to hang out. Those who suffer from headaches, insomnia, high or low blood pressure, destabilized knees, or sacroiliac or lower back problems should avoid this pose.

1. Reestablish slow and deep breaths through your nostrils.
2. Strengthen your exhalations by slowly contracting your abdominal muscles as you exhale. Do this without strain so the breath stays smooth.
3. Once you have comfortably established breathing with strong exhalations, add a brief pause at the end of each exhalation—just for a second or two—before starting your next inhalation. This technique stokes inner heat and stimulates metabolism.
4. Take a minute to establish this pattern of pausing for a moment at the end of each exhalation.
5. Make sure it's sustainable and you are not forcing or straining in any way. Use this breathing pattern throughout this next sequence.
6. Stand with your feet parallel, hip-width apart. Spread your toes wide and press firmly down through the soles of your feet.
7. Release your tailbone down while lifting your sternum and the crown of your head up.
8. Stand tall with your palms together at the center of your chest. Allow your shoulders to relax. Soften the muscles in the face, shoulders, and belly.
9. With your palms still touching, inhale your hands up and overhead.
10. Exhale your arms out to the sides and down as your knees bend and your hips hinge, coming into a squat (deep or shallow, whichever feels best).

11. Palms touch when you reach the bottom of the squat. Pause for a moment or two, suspending your breath, keeping your abdominals engaged.

12. Shift your weight back into your heels as you sink your hips down and lengthen your sternum up.

13. Inhale your hands up the centerline as your legs straighten and your arms reach overhead.

14. Exhale your arms out to the sides and down as your knees and hips bend, sinking into a squat. Palms touch. Pause with your breath held out and your belly engaged.

15. Inhale and draw your palms up the centerline, straightening your legs as your arms lift overhead.

16. Repeat, flowing with your breath—exhaling down into the squat, pausing with breath suspended, inhaling up to standing. The movement of the arms and legs will circulate energy.

17. Continue for five to ten rounds. Then release the movement and become still.

18. Let go of the breathing technique and breathe normally as you absorb the aftereffects of the pose.

Rhythmic Forward Fold
for Kapha

This pose will increase enthusiasm, improve digestion, and aid elimination by massaging and stimulating the abdominal organs, reducing your appetite, and expelling excess mucus via the force of gravity. Those who have uncontrolled high blood pressure or are pregnant or those with spinal issues such as herniated disc or sacroiliac problems should avoid this pose.

1. Stand with your feet parallel, hip-width distance apart.
2. Balance your weight evenly on your feet and firm them into the floor.
3. Stand tall by lifting the crown of your head up toward the ceiling. Inhale and float your arms up and overhead, with palms turned in and your fingers reaching up.
4. Exhale and draw your navel in and up as you fold forward from the hips, letting your knees bend slightly and your arms sweep down toward the floor and behind you.
5. Ground through your heels and lift your sitting bones toward the ceiling.
6. On an inhalation, sweep back up to standing as you lengthen the front of your torso, reaching your arms up and overhead.
7. Repeat the movement five to ten times.
8. Create a steady rhythm as you move with your breath, contracting your abdominals each time that you fold forward. Then return to standing.
9. Pause and take several breaths in stillness, feeling energy circulating through your body.

7

Energy Work

Assist the Flow of Prana

Prana is the life-force energy that flows through the body, called *chi* in Chinese medicine. One of the best ways help prana flow through the body is with yogic breathing, or pranayama. You'll notice that in yoga classes, pranayama (breath control) is an essential component, and that's because your breath is directly related to prana. By directing your breath, you direct your energy (prana), which boosts your stamina, energy, and focus. That flow of energy recharges your mind and body. See Breathwork (Chapter 4) for specific breathing exercises. Following are even easier ways to engage prana.

TWO SIMPLE WAYS TO FEEL PRANA

1. Notice how you feel mentally, emotionally, and physically, before your yoga practice, or before a nice, brisk walk outside. Then, after your practice (or your walk), take some time to notice any changes you feel in your mood or in your body. If you are feeling more balanced, more centered, and happier in mind and body, you're noticing the effect of prana flowing through the body and nourishing the cells.

2. Rub your hands together vigorously and breathe in and out three times, slowly. Gently separate your hands to create a small space between your palms. You will begin to feel sensation and pulsing in your hands. This is the sensation of prana moving.

Move That Body!

If a more stimulating shift of energy is what you need, bring more dance into your life. There are so many ways to bring dance into your life either with a guided CD or DVD, attending a class, or just listening to music and moving around the room. There isn't a right or wrong way to dance: Let the music be your body's guide.

If you aren't used to dancing or letting the music inform your movement, try this. When you turn on the music, even if it's fast-paced, close your eyes and pause. Wait a few moments to let the rhythm of the beat and the sounds affect your body; you don't have to think about it. And, then, after several moments, allow yourself to move in any way you like. The body knows what it needs; it will inform you. Again, do it with a light attitude—there's no one judging you. Smile as your body flows through space, and allow your mood to shift.

Get Moving with Your Children

Children can use the above tips just as adults can. Include your children in health-affirming exercises; this teaches them habits that they will have for their entire lives. For example, when you need to wind down before bed, include your children—teach them to wind down too. Model the behavior to them, even at times when they don't want to or won't cooperate. When you prioritize winding down, they will notice. Even if they don't respond right away, your actions will make an impression.

The same goes for doing yoga poses to take a pause in your day, or dancing around the room for stress relief and playfulness. Taking breaks is not a frivolous practice. There is time for focus, and there is time for play. The mind and body need breaks for restoration and proper functioning. Let your children see you and join you in creating that sense of balance in life.

Try a Walking Meditation

A walking meditation is a wonderful way to attune yourself to the rhythm and wisdom of the natural world. Your walking meditation takes you into the present moment, where you can allow other thoughts to drift by. It creates space and time for you to appreciate and connect to nature, which is so important for your understanding of yourself and the energy around you.

1. If it's cold outside wear enough layers to be warm. If it's hot out, be sure you can remove layers to be comfortable. Check the weather, so you can enjoy your walk.
2. After stepping outside, take a nice deep breath and let out a long exhalation. Do this a few times.
3. Set an intention for your walk. For example, "I'm taking a break now, there's no work for me to do on this walk. I can relax and be present to what is." Or, "I'm so grateful to live among such beauty, I'm going to spend some time appreciating it."
4. As you set out on your walk, intend to stop along the way, or before you turn around to come back. Use those pauses to notice the world around you. In the summer, stop to notice the details on the flowers, and see if a butterfly stops by. If it's wintertime, admire the translucence of icicles. Touch, smell, listen, and watch the world around you.
5. As other thoughts come to mind, allow them to be there. Then, bring your awareness back to exploring what's around you.
6. As you walk, when you're not admiring the changing natural world around you, notice how it feels when each foot touches the ground. Notice your posture. Notice how it feels to be bringing energy into the leg muscles. Swing the arms as you walk, get the bodily fluids flowing and pumping. Enjoy the movement.

7. When you've completed your walk, spend a moment in gratitude for that time outdoors. Allow that moment to be your acknowledgment of the good you've just done for your health.

Going on a walking meditation is healthy for your body, mind, and spirit. The mind gets a break, the body gets movement, and your spirit connects to the thriving life-force energy that's all around. If you go with your children, partner, or friend, remind each other of the beauty that surrounds you: the way the sun is hitting the trees, the sound of a bird that you can't see. What can you notice and share?

Brighten Your Mood

There are many things in life that can contribute to making you feel down. Everyone's life is full of waves: times when the ride feels smooth and times when the ride feels choppy. One of the best things you can do for your overall health is to learn ways to support yourself so that you can feel a sense of calm and contentment more often, even in the midst of many waves of energy. Of course, seek guidance from your doctors and Ayurvedic specialists so they can help you deal with your specific needs, especially if you are noticing your mood is often low and it's hard to feel content or at ease.

Food As Love and Comfort

Sometimes the phrase "comfort food" is thought of as bad for one's health. Often in the United States, "comfort food" seems to be thought of as the opposite to "healthy food." This is not necessarily true.

Instead of cutting out what you think of as comfort food, can you view more foods as comfort food? Can you begin to see anything you put into your body as comforting, nourishing, and worth smiling about? There's nothing wrong with eating and feeling comforted by the food you eat, when you eat well. Eating can boost your mood and make you feel better. Eating well makes it easier for you to see life clearly, be in the present moment, and think of ways to deal with life's challenges. According to Ayurveda, when you eat right for your type and in the right amount, food is medicine. It gives you mental and physical energy, and this will help stabilize mood swings. Even when you eat foods that cause imbalance, enjoy that food, too, as you eat it. It will make it easier to digest food well when you enjoy eating.

Also, hydrate yourself with warm water throughout the day, and control your portion size. Then you will find that eating what you need will make you feel very well. If you have been eating poorly for a while, it might take some time to get your body on track, and once you do, you will be able to brighten your mood by eating well. This supports your health and mood in the short and long run.

Feel Balanced, Graceful, and at Ease

Sometimes a mood brightener doesn't have to be something stimulating. Shifting your energy from a bit gloomy or a little frustrated can be as simple as a calming yoga posture known as Tree Pose. When you practice this pose you increase your focus, strength, balance, grace, and lightness. You also get blood moving in the body, which will really help your mood if you've been sitting for a while.

TREE POSE *(see image on page 7 of the insert)*

1. Come into standing, and hold on to the back of a chair if you need to, for balance.
2. Feel your feet rooting into the earth. Engage the leg muscles, and feel your spine elongate as you imagine the crown of your head lifting toward the ceiling.
3. Exhale, and shift your weight onto the left leg; notice how solid and sturdy that leg is.
4. Inhale, engage the abdomen muscles, and lift the right foot off the floor and place your right foot against your left knee to make a triangle. Keep your pelvis facing forward. If you can't comfortably lift your foot all the way to your knee, do not push it. Simply rest it against your calf.
5. Breathe normally, and fix your gaze on a point in front of you. Keep your gaze steady and soft.
6. Bring your awareness to the strength of the left leg, the softness of your gaze, and the joy of balancing.
7. Bring your hands straight up over your head. Breathe in and out for several breaths. Bring your hands straight up over your head.
8. Replace the right foot on the ground.

After doing Tree Pose, notice how you feel. Do you notice a difference in one side of the body or the other? After pausing to notice the effects of Tree Pose, do the pose on the other side.

When you do Tree Pose, be light about it. It isn't a contest. If you can't stay balanced, it's okay. If it's not easy the first time or second time, it's okay; it will get easier. The goal is to practice coming to the pose with ease and lightness of spirit. And, with time, your balance will likely increase, and you'll be able to do the pose with more ease and lightness.

Tree Pose is something you and your children can do together. Increase the imagery when you do it. Talk about seeing the water around you, the colors of the sunrise in front you, etc.

Five-Minute Mood Changers

If you're feeling heavy and unmotivated, see if you can take a five-minute break to do something special for yourself to switch your mood. Here are some ideas:

- **Make a cup of tea.** There are so many varieties of tea, and many companies are making their teas in transparent tea bags with wonderfully fresh and innovative blends inside. Once you find out what teas you like, keep some in your office and home. And when you need a pick-me-up, take a tea break to shift your mood.

- **Stop what you're doing (or not doing), and write down something that you'd rather be doing instead,** whether it's being with your children, going to a movie, or going to the beach. Make it simple, and also something you'd really like to do. Then write down the steps you have to take to make it happen. Resolve to find time to do each step, as you can.

- **Stand up and shake it off.** Stand up where you are and feel your feet firmly on the ground. Then lift one foot at a time and shake your leg while you inhale and exhale three times. (If balancing is hard for you, hold on to the back of a chair so you don't fall.) After you shake out both legs, shake out your arms for three long breaths.

Sometimes the best thing you can do is make a momentary shift in what you're doing, and that can change your mood.

Learn about Marma Therapy

Marmas are sensitive energetic zones in and on the body. *Marma* means "vulnerable" or "sensitive." You can use marma therapy to facilitate the flow of prana or to stop the flow of prana at particular sites on the body. In other words, you can focus on marma points to heal a person's ailments, and you could use them to end a person's life. The marma points are taught to students of martial arts (for self-defense), and they are taught to students of Ayurveda and yoga as powerful sites that can set deep healing in motion.

Where Are Marmas?

The major Ayurvedic texts list 51 marma regions and 107 marma points. (The number of points is greater than the number of regions because some regions have more than one point, and also to reach some regions there is a point on the back of the body and the front of the body.) Marmas cover the entire body, and many Ayurvedic teachers recognize more than 107 marma points.

The ancient texts list specific places where you can find marmas throughout the body, but remember that Ayurveda acknowledges everyone as an individual. The exact location of marmas will be different (at least slightly) for each person. When sending healing energy to the body, the prana will find its way into the places where prana is very low. Just as water flows toward where there is space, prana flows to where it's needed. The points listed in the textbooks are useful as a guide, a point of departure and understanding. The interaction between the healer and the patient will reveal where the most sensitive spots are for that person.

Marmas and the Doshas

Marma therapy can be used for all doshas, and can treat a variety of imbalances that are associated with particular doshas. For vata dosha, marma therapy can have many balancing effects, including:

○ Relieving pain in bones and joints
○ Calming anxiety
○ Promoting sleep
○ Relieving constipation

For pitta dosha, again, there are many benefits, which include:

○ Calming anger
○ Reducing acidity in small intestine
○ Cleansing the blood

Marma therapy can relieve kapha symptoms, including:

○ Increasing mental and physical energy
○ Clearing mucus
○ Stimulating weight loss

All Ayurvedic therapies benefit from the knowledge of marma therapy because it works directly with prana in the body. Using the marma points correctly, you can increase or decrease heat in the body, as well as address long-term and degenerative disease.

You can also use knowledge of marma points to understand your own energy body. It can help you in your yoga practice and with your self-massage. One thorough guide for learning the placement of the marmas and how to work with them is *Ayurveda and Marma Therapy* by Dr. David Frawley, Dr. Subhash Ranade, and Dr. Avinash Lele.

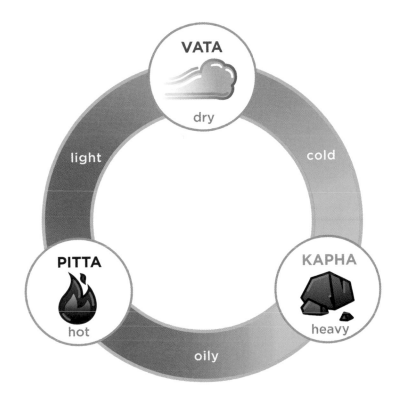

Ayurveda assesses your state of being and the state of the natural world in terms of three basic principles, or *doshas*. The doshas are vata, pitta, and kapha. Vata is a combination of the elements ether and air, pitta is a combination of fire and water, and kapha is both water and earth elements.

Image by Eric Andrews

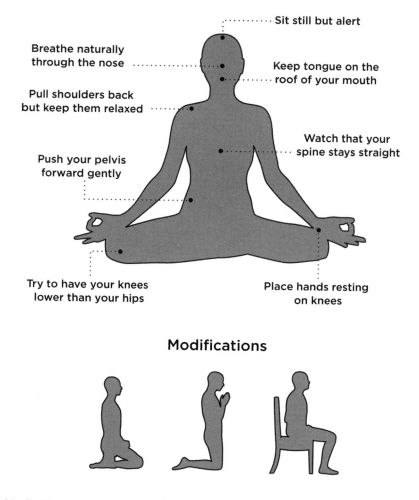

Sit still but alert

Breathe naturally through the nose

Keep tongue on the roof of your mouth

Pull shoulders back but keep them relaxed

Watch that your spine stays straight

Push your pelvis forward gently

Try to have your knees lower than your hips

Place hands resting on knees

Modifications

Meditation is the practice of detaching from ongoing trains of thought, or the practice of focusing on a specific object such as a mantra or image. It's one of the many therapies used in Ayurveda because it helps you find mental clarity and equilibrium. These postures will help your body achieve calmness and balance.

Images by Eric Andrews

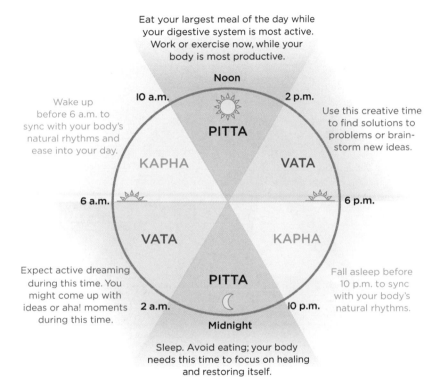

Eat your largest meal of the day while your digestive system is most active. Work or exercise now, while your body is most productive.

Wake up before 6 a.m. to sync with your body's natural rhythms and ease into your day.

Noon

10 a.m.

2 p.m.

PITTA

KAPHA

VATA

Use this creative time to find solutions to problems or brainstorm new ideas.

6 a.m.

6 p.m.

VATA

KAPHA

Expect active dreaming during this time. You might come up with ideas or aha! moments during this time.

PITTA

2 a.m.

10 p.m.

Midnight

Fall asleep before 10 p.m. to sync with your body's natural rhythms.

Sleep. Avoid eating; your body needs this time to focus on healing and restoring itself.

The daily cycle of the Ayurvedic clock helps you understand when it's best to wake up (before kapha time), when to eat your biggest meal (lunchtime, pitta time), and what time to go to sleep (before pitta time) based on the qualities associated with each dosha.

Image by Eric Andrews

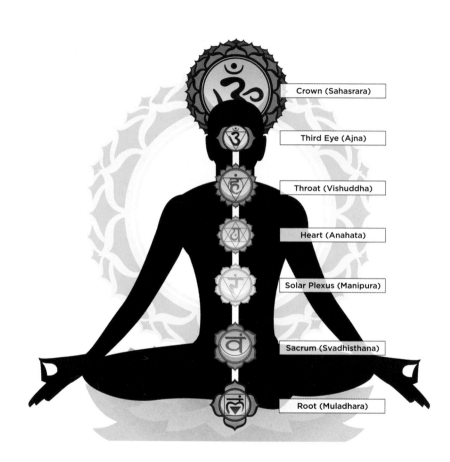

Crown (Sahasrara)

Third Eye (Ajna)

Throat (Vishuddha)

Heart (Anahata)

Solar Plexus (Manipura)

Sacrum (Svadhisthana)

Root (Muladhara)

There are seven major chakras in the body. They are like conductors of energy, and their balance or imbalance affects your overall health.

Image © Getty Images/Tomacco

4

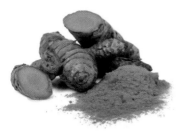

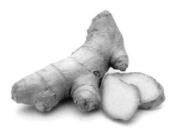

Turmeric is an anti-inflammatory that is great for alleviating symptoms of colds and flus. It is also an astringent flavor you can use to balance your dosha via nutritional intake.

Image © Getty Images/lathuric

Ginger can help you fight colds and flus, plus it is well known for its abilities to calm the digestive system. It's also a pungent flavor.

Image © Getty Images/Natikka

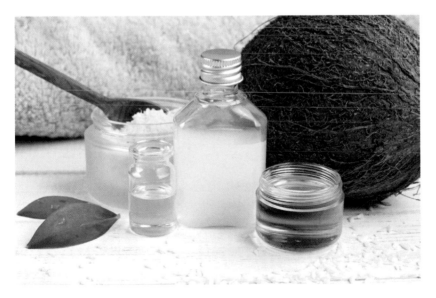

Self-massage with warm oil is a great way to prepare your body for sleep.

Image © Getty Images/Anna-Ok

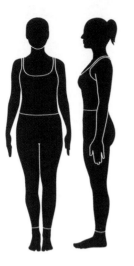

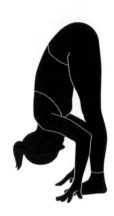

Mountain Pose for VATA and KAPHA
This majestic stretch helps balance vata within the abdominal area and also helps kapha types start their day.

Standing Forward Fold for KAPHA This stretch also strengthens many areas of the body.

Warrior I Pose for VATA and KAPHA This pose helps balance vata by stretching the pelvic area and the lower abdomen, and nourishes and balances the endocrine, circulatory, respiratory, digestive, and immune systems for kapha types.

Images by Eric Andrews

Plank Pose for KAPHA Strengthen your exhalations in this pose by drawing your navel back toward your spine as you breathe out.

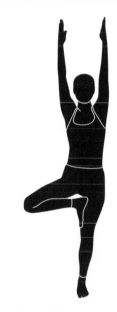

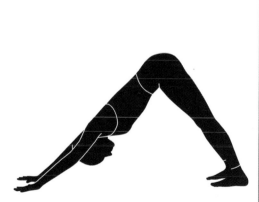

Downward Facing Dog for KAPHA Breathing deeply in this pose helps activate the respiratory system.

Images by Eric Andrews

Tree Pose This lengthening pose helps stimulate the circulatory system and promote balance and focus.

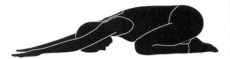

Child's Pose for VATA Feel the earth grounding and supporting you at all the points where you're touching the ground.

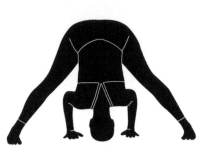

Standing Wide-Angle Forward Fold for PITTA This pose circulates abdominal energy, calms an overheated brain, and helps dispel excess heat.

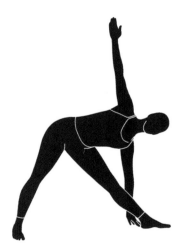

Twisting Wide-Angle Forward Fold for PITTA This twist helps wring out excess heat, which balances pitta.

Images by Eric Andrews

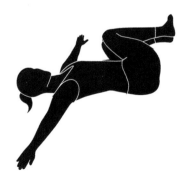

Reclined Twist for PITTA This twist is great for pitta types because it's calming and not overly heating.

✳

Practice Hand Mudras

Another very effective and creative way to move energy through the body is to use hand mudras, or postures for the hands. This also can be practiced with children because it's fun to hold the hands in different positions and envision the energy flowing through the body.

> **MUDRAS ARE VERSATILE**
> You don't have to be sitting to use mudras. You can stand, walk, or even dance while you hold your hands in specific postures. Bringing joy and creativity to energetic healing makes it a special addition to your day, rather than something you feel you have to do.

Each mudra is used for a particular purpose. The way you hold your hands activates different marmas and also directs energy to different parts of the body.

Hand Mudra for Inner Harmony

In her book *Mudras: Yoga in Your Hands*, Gertrud Hirschi explains how to do a variety of mudras. This posture, Matangi, is for inner harmony and rulership.

MATANGI MUDRA
1. Bring the palms of the hands together.
2. With fingers and palms touching, spread the fingers.
3. Fold the fingers of the right and left hand all the way down, so you interlace the fingers.
4. With the fingers of the hands interlaced and folded down, extend the two middle fingers up, and allow them to press against each other.
5. Hold for several breaths, then release the posture.

According to Hirschi, you should do this posture as needed or three times per day for four minutes. This mudra brings balance to the solar plexus, to the heart, and to the process of digestion. All of these benefits enhance your Ayurvedic lifestyle.

In addition, this mudra stimulates the earth element, which is an element of kapha. So, it will help ground vata and pitta, and bring some extra support to kapha. All of the doshas can use the pranic support that this mudra sends to the regions of the body and to the process of digestion.

Hand Mudra to Help Energy Flow in Joints

Joint pain is often called "chronic" and can especially affect those with vata imbalance. Having a mudra that you can practice is an easy option to help energy flow. You do have to be diligent with it. Hirschi recommends holding this posture four times a day for fifteen minutes each time. She also recommends that if there is illness, you should hold the mudra twice as long, six times per day.

MUDRA TO RELIEVE JOINT PAIN
1. Open the right hand, and touch the thumb to the ring finger.
2. Open the left hand and touch the thumb to the middle finger.
3. Hold both hands like this, and breathe normally. Envision and enjoy the healing flow of energy.

Mudras, like other yoga poses and other forms of energetic healing, may take some time to work. Sometimes you'll feel immediate relief, other times you may not. Some of the benefits of doing mudras (rather than taking over-the-counter or prescription drugs) are that mudras are all natural, there are no side effects, you will not become physically dependent on them, and they are free!

8

Healing

⁕

Fight Colds

When you notice a cold coming on, start to support your body in clearing out the mucus and irritants. Be sure you are hydrating yourself well, and get extra rest. One way to prevent colds is to keep your immune system strong by keeping yourself balanced as best as you can. Then you will either avoid catching colds altogether, or when you do catch one it will be much easier to treat.

Turmeric for Colds

Turmeric *(see image on page 5 of the insert)* is an anti-inflammatory that can help clear excess mucus (for children and adults alike). One way to take turmeric is to make a paste of equal parts turmeric and raw honey. Begin by taking one tablespoon of this mixture every hour for the first few hours, and then reduce the frequency to once about every four to six hours. If symptoms do not improve after the first day, talk to your doctor.

You can also add turmeric to your diet on a regular basis, and not wait until you catch a cold. It's a delicious seasoning to add to rice, pasta, and vegetables any time of year. For a more complex taste, mix it with other spices to create a curry powder.

Ginger for Colds and Flu

An excellent ingredient for combating a cold or flu is ginger. The extra mucus your body creates comes from excess kapha, and it's possible that vata will be in excess as well when you have a cold or flu—leading to chills and poor appetite.

Ginger is hot, pungent, and stimulating, which is great for countering the effects of too much kapha and vata. In *The Complete Book of Ayurvedic Home Remedies*, Dr. Vasant Lad gives a simple recipe for a ginger brew to take several times a day when you have a cold or flu:

GINGER BREW

1. Combine ginger, cinnamon, and lemongrass in the ratio 1:1:2, or substitute a pinch of cardamom for the lemongrass.
2. Steep this mixture in hot water for ten minutes, then strain.
3. If you'd like to add sweetness, use honey.

You can make an even simpler brew by steeping only freshly grated ginger in boiling water. After about ten minutes, drink and savor the healing effects of ginger.

> SAFETY NOTE
>
> Do not take aspirin and ginger at the same time; they both thin the blood. Take them at least two hours apart, if you want to take them both. Because of the dangers of improper food, herb, and medicine combinations, get advice from your specialist before trying remedies that are new to you at home.

Steaming

Steaming is a fast and effective way to deal with congestion, sore throat, and runny nose. You can simply pour boiling water into a bowl, then hold your head over the bowl with a towel over your head to keep the steam in. Close your eyes and breathe deeply.

Spend about ten to fifteen minutes inhaling the steam. You can do this several times a day.

You can steam with plain water, or add a drop of eucalyptus essential oil or tea tree essential oil to the bowl after you've poured the boiling water into it. These herbs are naturally antiseptic. Inhale the steam nice and deeply into the sinuses, back of the throat, and lungs.

Use Abhyanga

By using the wisdom of Ayurveda, you can keep colds and flu from entering the house and making the rounds, family member by family member. One of the best things to begin with is the practice of abhyanga, herbalized-oil massage. On top of having many important health benefits, abhyanga feels luxurious. The primary benefits of abhyanga are:

- Keeps the skin moisturized, preventing eczema and rash
- Supports the lymphatic system, which is how the body collects and removes pollutants
- Induces the feeling of being supported, balanced, and relaxed

Each of those benefits significantly supports the entire person: psychologically, physically, and energetically. In particular, oiling the skin has a direct effect on the lymphatic system, which is your body's way of capturing and removing the pollutants that can lead to allergies, colds, and flu. The oil penetrates into the deeper tissues, keeping them lubricated and able to support the various functions of the body, including the elimination of waste.

How and When to Do Abhyanga

Do abhyanga before entering the bath or shower in the morning. It's especially soothing to warm the oil first, by running the bottle under warm water. Then, as you massage the oil into your skin (or your child's), massage in long strokes along the limbs, and massage in circular motions over the joints. Be sure to massage the entire body, in loving strokes. This includes massaging oil into the scalp. Once your children are old enough, they can do abhyanga without your help. Learning to self-nuture is a wonderful skill for them to take into adulthood. If your child is predominantly vata, or has a vata imbalance, it will help to give her a soothing foot massage with oil before she goes to bed.

Minimize Bloating

When you have gas, allow yourself to release it from the body as flatulence or burping. Gas in the colon is considered an excess of vata, and holding it in will create more vata disturbance in the body.

Pacify Vata

If you're feeling the pain of gas in the colon often, and you have a lot of flatulence, try a vata-pacifying diet. This will help bring moisture and heaviness into your body, to balance the winds of vata.

Also, when you perform your daily self-massage, make sure you are oiling your torso well. Gently massage the area of your torso where the colon is, bringing your awareness and care to that area of the body: back and front.

Regulate Your Elimination

Sometimes gas builds up in conjunction with constipation, another sign of vata imbalance. You can regulate your elimination by taking triphala. Take a tablet with a glass of water, or boil a teaspoon of the powdered form in water. Take triphala before going to bed. It's a mild herb, suitable for all doshas, so you can take it regularly for four to six weeks.

A Mixture to Take after Meals

Try this spice mixture to ease gas. Roast cumin, coriander, and ajwan seeds separately for one to three minutes in a dry pan (stir to prevent burning). When done, remove them from the heat and mix together. After each meal, put about a teaspoon of the mixture in your mouth, chew it well, then wash it down with warm water.

Another option to help digestion is to make a ginger tea. You can sip the tea on an empty stomach or drink it about a half hour before meals.

Relieve Lower Back Pain

Low back pain can be caused by several factors, emotional as well as physical. Certain home remedies can help, though serious injuries (like a slipped disc) will require professional medical attention and supervision.

Remedies for Lower Back Pain

When you have lower back pain, or any back pain, your Ayurvedic specialist may recommend certain herbs to help relax the muscles. You also can rub mahanarayan oil on the affected area and take a hot bath; or lie down in a comfortable position and try this visualization:

1. Lie down in a comfortable position. If you're on your back, place a pillow or two underneath your knees. If you're curled up on your side, place a pillow in between your knees. See if those pillows make the posture more comfortable.
2. Envision the muscles of the back relaxing into the support of the floor beneath you.
3. Take deep nourishing breaths; on each inhalation envision your breath carrying healing life-force energy to the entire back, especially the area that hurts.
4. On each exhalation, envision exhaling any emotional and physical pain.
5. After several rounds of deep breaths, return to normal breathing. Envision relaxing the entire body.

When you're ready to sit up after this visualization, sit up very slowly. There's no rush.

The benefits of learning to relax and let go cannot be overstated. Your mind and body need time to restore, relax, and rejuvenate. Stress is often cited as the cause of imbalance and illness. Practice letting it all go.

Pacify Vata

Because the colon is located in the same region of the body as the lower back, disturbances in vata can cause low back pain. If you experience lower back pain, follow a vata-pacifying diet, keep yourself warm, surround yourself with calming friends and family, and create routine when you can—at the very least, at mealtimes and bedtime. As you start to pacify vata, you will help support the relaxation of the back.

Kati Basti

A wonderfully soothing and healing procedure, Kati Basti is used for various types of back pain and discomfort from sciatica to herniated discs. To do this, you will lie down on your belly, and a trained practitioner will make a circular flour dam on your back. Then, he will pour warm herbalized oil inside the dam. You will relax for several minutes while the warm, medicated oil sinks into your skin and into the body.

THE POWER OF VISUALIZATION

Visualizations are very powerful healing tools. When you're experiencing any kind of pain in the body, visualize health and comfort where you feel pain. Place your hand on that body part, too, if you can reach it. The visualization will let your body know you are responding to its "alarm signal," which is what pain is.

Treat Acne

Acne can be the result of emotional, hormonal, or bacterial causes. It's important to find out what the cause is, so it can be properly treated. By all accounts, whatever the root cause, it signifies aggravated pitta. Pitta moves under the skin and then erupts as acne (or rash, hives, eczema, etc.).

Pacify Pitta

Follow a pitta-pacifying diet. Also, don't spend time playing outside in extremely hot weather: If you want to be outside, be sure it's not during the hottest hours of the day. Practice pitta-pacifying yoga, meditation, and breathwork.

Put Your Mind on Something Else

If you worry and stress about your acne, it will likely not disappear. The key is to relax and pacify pitta as often as you can in your life. So, if you start to become worried or unhappy, try to turn your attention to something that is calming and relaxing in your life. When you do think of your skin, imagine it as clear, and then take your mind off it. Take a walk outside or listen to some music that you enjoy. Learning to relax and calm the mind and body will be effective, whereas continuing to think about the acne will aggravate it.

Prevent Insomnia

There are a number of remedies you can try to help with trouble falling asleep and staying asleep. One thing to start doing is to avoid stimulating activites starting at least one hour before bed. That means no television, no computer, and no overly stimulating reading material. Do relaxing activities like listening to soothing music, reading books that aren't disturbing, or listening to a yoga nidra CD. You can take a warm bath, do a self-massage, or sit outside and look at the stars.

Soothing Drinks

Make yourself a cup of warm milk. Add spice to it such as a teaspoon of turmeric, a teaspoon of nutmeg, and a teaspoon of cinnamon. Add ½ tablespoon of ghee, and you've got yourself a soothing bedtime drink.

If you don't like milk, you can also enjoy a cup of chamomile tea or peppermint tea before bed. When you prepare yourself a calming drink before bed, keep your attention on enjoying the beverage and noticing the quiet of nighttime. Allow yourself to sink into the peacefulness of the night and the warmth of the drink. Slowly take sips, and notice how it makes you feel. Don't watch television or do stimulating activities: That counteracts the effect.

Oil the Feet

A self-massage before bed is a relaxing way to transition from an active mind to a body ready for rest. It's especially effective to massage your feet with oil, slowly, rhythmically, and with mindfulness. Take your time as you rub oil into the soles and heels of your feet. Pay special attention to the toes. Wind down with this nourishing bedtime ritual.

Stop Nosebleeds

According to Dr. Lad, nosebleeds are considered pitta. To balance the heat, use cooling remedies to effectively stop a nosebleed. There can be many causes, and as with all symptoms, if some simple remedies do not help, you must see a doctor. While many nosebleeds can be simple to stop because they are from dryness in the nasal passages, allergies, or stress, some nosebleeds can be caused by more serious conditions. If after trying several remedies the nosebleed doesn't stop, see a doctor.

If You Have a Nosebleed, Relax

One of the most important things you can do, especially while doing these recommended remedies, is relax. Nosebleeds can be aggravated by stress. Stand or sit up (lying down can cause more bleeding), and relax. Breathe deep into the belly to help encourage the relaxation response. Relax.

Use Cold Water

To stop a nosebleed, it will help to cool the nose and cool yourself internally to balance pitta. Try these methods:

1. Drink a glass of cool water.
2. Rinse a clean washcloth in cool water, and use it as a compress for the forehead and nose.
3. Very gently blow the nose to get out any obstruction that may be causing the nosebleed, then place a cube of ice (wrapped in a towel) on the side of the nose that is bleeding.

Each of these options is very cooling, so even just doing one usually will stop a nosebleed.

Other Remedies to Try

If cooling the nose and body isn't enough to stop the nosebleed, pinch the nose for a few moments. Don't tilt your head back, just pinch the nose. Usually after three to five minutes the bleeding will stop.

GHEE ISN'T JUST FOR EATING!
Ghee to the rescue again! Ghee is hemostatic; it stops bleeding. Warm up some ghee and put a few drops into the nose if other methods aren't working. You can also put some ghee on a cotton swab and carefully swab inside the nostrils. Be gentle; you don't need to cause more irritation in the nose.

Pomegranate and cranberry juices can also stop nosebleeds. You can both drink the juice, and put a few drops into the nose to stop bleeding.

Prevent Nosebleeds

After you've stopped the nosebleed, do what you can to prevent nosebleeds by keeping yourself well hydrated and making sure the rooms in your home and in your office have enough humidity (using a hot water humidifier). Also, if you use a neti pot each day or at least oil your nasal passages each day, this will help keep the nasal passages clear, clean, and lubricated.

Monitoring your stress levels will also help. Before bedtime each night, take at least five to ten minutes to just pause and do nothing. Just sit still and consciously relax the body. To do this you can try this exercise:

FIVE-MINUTE RELAXATION BEFORE BED

1. Sit upright at the edge of the bed, or in the bed, if this is comfortable for you. If lying down is more comfortable, do so. Do not go straight to sleep.

2. As you are sitting or lying down, close your eyes. Feel the heaviness of the eyelids; notice how closing the eyes helps you shut out the distractions of the day.

3. Notice your breath; take a few deep breaths in, and long exhalations out. Then, return to normal breathing.
4. Gently give yourself a soothing face massage. In a slow and methodical way, rub away tension from your forehead, your temples, your jawline, and then any part of your body that needs some attention.

When you're finished, slowly slide into the bed for sleeping. Move at a slow pace; encourage a restful transition from using your senses all day. Keeping yourself relaxed and hydrated could be all you need to prevent future nosebleeds.

Soothe Indigestion

Indigestion can be caused by many factors, so talk to your Ayurvedic specialist and determine what is causing it for you. Once you get to the root of the indigestion, you will be able to prevent it. You and your specialist will be able to determine if you are experiencing vata, pitta, or kapha indigestion. Talking with her and dealing with the doshic imbalance will have long-term effects, which is better than dealing with indigestion only when it happens.

Helping Digestion with Ginger

Once you are feeling indigestion, it is likely caused by low digestive fire. Drinking a cup of ginger tea a half hour before meals is a great way to stoke the digestive fire. If you initiate your digestive fire this way before eating, you help your body prepare to digest food.

Another way to take ginger *(see image on page 5 of the insert)* is to simply chew fresh ginger. Cut a thin slice of ginger and chew on it. Allow the taste and the juice to prepare your body for digestion.

> **SLOW DOWN**
> When you are experiencing indigestion, don't eat if you aren't hungry. Give your system some time to work out what's going on, and relax as best as you can. According to Ayurveda it's always best not to eat if you aren't hungry.

Peppermint for Bellyache

Peppermint can be very soothing to the gut, especially if you're experiencing acidity in the digestive tract. Make peppermint tea by boiling water and pouring it over loose-leaf peppermint. Allow it to steep for ten minutes. Sip slowly and become aware of the aroma and the taste of the peppermint as it goes to the site to relieve your discomfort.

Peppermint is a wonderful herb for balance in summertime. If you grow it outside, or buy it fresh, try smelling it (without ingesting) and notice the cooling effect on your emotions and mental state. Your sense of smell is the only sense pathway that goes straight to the limbic system—the part of the brain that experiences emotions.

Soothing the Belly with Your Healing Hands

If you are experiencing pain with indigestion, give your belly a gentle and comforting massage. Rub your belly in a clockwise motion, going up the right side of the body, across the top of where the colon is, and down the left side. Repeat this for several rounds. As you do this, inhale and exhale deeply, bringing soothing energy to your digestive tract.

After doing this in the front, place your hand on your lower back—the other side of where your digestive organs reside. Send healing energy for several breaths through the back side of your body.

✳
Using Gems for Healing

Ayurvedic wisdom teaches about healing properties in gems. The following are general guidelines about gems. In general, it's important for you to talk to someone who is well trained in this aspect of Ayurveda for the most effective advice about what would be most supportive to you. When you talk to a specialist, he can help make sure you choose the right gems, that you wear them on the appropriate finger (or as a necklace), and that you choose an appropriate setting.

The Healing Power of Gems

Like all things of nature, gems carry energy. Gem therapy is energetic therapy—energy from the gem interacts with your energy field. Gems help support you with energy that you need, where you are deficient.

Many gems will absorb the energy around them, so it's important to cleanse your gems before you use them or wear them. After they are cleansed, they are restored with their own healing energy, and any other energy they may have picked up has been washed away.

> **CLEANSING GEMS**
>
> To cleanse a gem that is not water-soluble, find a spring or another type of natural water source. Bring your gem to the natural water source, and rinse it under the fresh water for a few moments. Pull the gem out of the water, and state your healing intentions.

Each gem has energy that heals a particular aspect of you. See the following table, which shows how Ayurveda categorizes the gems.

Gem	Uses
Diamond	imagination, love
Emerald	perception, discernment
Pearl	mental calm, serenity
Red Coral	vitality
Ruby	self-esteem
Sapphire (blue)	independence, patience
Sapphire (yellow)	wisdom, creativity

For less expensive versions of the above gems try:

- Clear quartz for diamond
- Jade for emerald
- Moonstone for pearl
- Garnet for ruby
- Lapis lazuli for blue sapphire
- Citrine for yellow sapphire

There are other gems, too, with additional healing properties. For as many conditions as the human body can exhibit, there are gems to help. Your specialist in Vedic astrology, *jyotish*, will be able to guide you.

Gems can also be used because of how they affect doshas in you. Based on the energies of the planets, certain gems will balance or aggravate certain doshas. For example, blue sapphire calms vata and kapha, and opal calms pitta.

Aside from wearing gems, you can also make water infused with their healing energy. To do this, place a flawless gem in clear, spring water overnight. The next day, sip the water to receive the benefits. The water will be energized with the healing qualities of that gem. This is a great way to receive energy from gems in the meantime, before talking to a specialist for more specific advice that is personalized for you.

PART III

A Lifetime of Balance

9

Visits with an Ayurvedic Practitioner or Consultant

The Questionnaire

Visits with an Ayurvedic practitioner help you feel empowered. During your visit, she will ask about a variety of aspects of your life, including the symptoms or ailments you are presenting. By answering her questions, you'll tell her how you are holding up psychologically, physically, and energetically, so she can make natural and holistic suggestions for your overall healing. Her recommendations will help you understand what you need, and why, to deal with your present symptoms and get on the path to long-term health.

Before visiting your Ayurvedic specialist, you will fill out a questionnaire. The questionnaire will give your practitioner information about your health history and how you are feeling now. The questionnaire is likely different from what you experience with most Western doctors because it's designed to give a full picture of how you are living your life, not only focusing on disease or pain.

Topics Covered in the Questionnaire

Not all questionnaires from Ayurvedic practitioners will be the same, but they will generally cover the same topics. Here are some areas of your life the questionnaire will cover:

- Your family's health history
- Your present symptoms and their duration
- What medications you're taking (if any)
- Your eating, sleeping, and exercise habits
- What tastes you crave
- The frequency and qualities of your elimination (stool and urine)
- Your energy level

The specific questions will guide you toward painting a full picture of your lifestyle and habits. For example, regarding your sleeping habits, they will want to know what time you go to bed, what time you typically wake up, whether your sleep is heavy, if you have nightmares, and whether you wake up refreshed.

Something unique about the Ayurvedic questionnaire is that it will ask how you would describe your family life, social life, work life, and spiritual life. Your relationship to these components of your life can affect your health, and also can give your practitioner more information about your prakruti and vikruti.

BE HONEST

When filling out the Ayurvedic questionnaire, do your best to answer the questions as truthfully as you can. It is suggested to answer the questions by looking at yourself through time from childhood to present and answering from what has been most consistent in your nature over time, and most especially how it showed up in childhood.

What You Can Learn from the Questionnaire

There are no "right" or "wrong" answers to the questions. They are designed to help your practitioner gauge how you are and what kinds of changes could support your healing and continued health.

The questionnaire is designed to help your practitioner understand various aspects of your life, and you, too, can learn a lot about yourself and your lifestyle as you fill it out. In this way, the questionnaire is a guide that helps you learn what to notice about yourself. It may present questions about your diet or lifestyle that you never thought to notice, and so now you can take the time to notice and your practitioner can help you make healthier choices.

Pulse Diagnosis

Your Ayurvedic specialist will be able to understand a lot about the health of your body by reading your pulse. Pulse diagnosis is a foundational, intricate, and unique aspect of Ayurveda. Modern Western doctors also use the pulse as a means for determining certain health factors, but Ayurveda uses it in a more detailed way to discover much more about what's going on with your body, mind, and energy flow.

Feeling and Listening to the Doshas

Your Ayurvedic practitioner will use your pulse to discover many things about your health, including how the doshas are showing up in you. The pulse diagnosis is the way your practitioner can really listen to what your body has to say and tune in to how your life force is flowing.

Ayurveda contains extensive instruction and wisdom about the various aspects of health that a practitioner can determine from the pulse. It takes practice, study, and sensitivity to be able to interpret the numerous types of messages that the pulse contains. In keeping with its connection to nature, Ayurveda uses animals as metaphors for how the pulse moves. Vata in balance feels like the movement of a cobra, pitta in balance hops like a frog, and kapha in balance glides like a swan.

There are various parts of the body where you can have your pulse taken. Often the radial pulse, near the wrist, is a common place to read the pulse.

What Advanced Practitioners Can Determine

With study and practice, a well-trained, skilled, and sensitive practitioner can use pulse diagnosis to determine the condition of your doshas and much more. The pulse diagnosis is an important part of the visit between you and your practitioner. It helps support and add important information to the other components of her evaluation.

Your Physical Appearance and the Doshas

Your internal world and external appearance are connected. What's happening inside of you, mentally, energetically, and physically, will show in your physical appearance. When it comes to the doshas, the way the qualities of the elements are acting in you will cause certain signs in your physical appearance. Your Ayurvedic practitioner can notice qualities in your physical appearance that reflect qualities associated with vata, pitta, and kapha.

Vata

Signs of strong vata are dry and brittle nails and hair. A person of vata constitution will usually have small eyes. He will have a thin body frame, and skin that is dry and rough.

If you think about the qualities of vata—dry, rough, and cold—then it makes sense that the physical qualities associated with vata would be dry hair, nails, and skin. The qualities of air and space in the body make it thin, brittle, and dry.

Pitta

A person exhibiting pitta qualities will have penetrating eyes, usually green or gray. Her nails will be healthy and smooth. Her body's frame will be of moderate size, her skin oily and warm, and she'll easily perspire. Her hair could be red, and go to gray early. She may have freckles, on her fair, red, or yellowish skin.

With the elements of pitta being of both fire and water, pitta's outward show is wet, hot, and sharp. And those qualities will show up in the hair, nails, skin, and other body parts.

Kapha

Kapha's eyes are large, round, and have thick eyelashes. The nails are thick and strong. A kapha's body type is large and round, and his skin is oily and pale. His hair could be thick and oily, and his teeth strong and white.

Kapha is a combination of earth and water, so thick, heavy, and wet qualities will show up outwardly. Coolness is also associated with kapha, so kapha's skin may be cool to the touch.

Tongue

The tongue is an important part of your digestive process. It helps move food around in your mouth so you can chew it, and it provides saliva to help break down food. The tongue is also an indicator of how well you are digesting and absorbing nutrients.

TALES OF THE TONGUE

When you stick out your tongue, if you notice that it trembles or is shaky, that's a sign that you're experiencing fear and/or a fair amount of stress. Take a moment now, and see if your tongue is shaky when you stick it out. If so, is it accurately reflecting that you feel fear or stress? By looking at your tongue, your practitioner will be able to realize how your colon and small intestines are doing, as well as other parts of your body, including your heart, spine, lungs, and kidneys.

There are many more evaluations your practitioner will be able to make based on these and other aspects of your physical appearance. Ayurveda is a vast science, and your outward appearance can reveal so much about your internal state of being because you are a whole, interconnected being. What goes on for you internally will reflect externally.

Sitting Down for a Heart-to-Heart

Ayurveda puts great emphasis on your emotions, thoughts, and beliefs because they all influence your health. Love and kindness are healing. When you go in to visit with your Ayurvedic practitioner, you are entering a place where he will see you as a full being. He will not just be looking at your symptoms and their biological functions. He will be sitting with you, listening to you, talking to you, and wanting to assess how the various aspects of your life combine together and determine how you are feeling now. You can come to the meeting with the intention of openhearted and safe discussion, where you are being seen as a total and unique person.

Taking Your Time

As your Ayurvedic practitioner asks you questions, you can take a moment to think about the answer. Sometimes it might take you some time to think about an aspect of your life you haven't been noticing or thinking about. So don't feel you have to say the first thing that comes to mind. Giving accurate information is more important than rushing.

As you meet with your consultant, ask questions if there's something you don't understand. When you go home later to follow his advice, it will help if you understand why you are doing what you are doing. Your understanding and visualizations of the healing process really do support its efficacy. You are a key participant in your healing process, and your Ayurvedic practitioner provides his expertise and guidance to help you along the way.

New Topics on the Table

When you talk with your Ayurvedic practitioner, you may find yourself discussing topics that you aren't used to having on the table with doctors. The topics will include your elimination, your diet, your relationships, and your work life. These could feel like personal topics, and you may not be used to discussing them with your doctors.

JUST BE

When talking to your practitioner, try to let go of any judgment you have about your health. If you have diarrhea, your tongue is coated with a white film, and/or your nails are brittle, allow all of that to be the truth, without judgment. Just notice how you are, and cultivate compassion for your body and all it's coping with.

There's good reason for why a variety of subjects will come up when you talk with your Ayurvedic specialist. Hearing about the various components of your life informs your practitioner about how the doshas are working in you and how your environment might be affecting you. From there, he can give sound advice about how to create balance, good digestion, and lasting health.

The Recommendations You Can Expect

When you visit with your Ayurvedic specialist, he'll ask about your lifestyle and diet before making recommendations for your health. Specifically, some of the topics he'll be most interested in discussing are your eating and sleeping habits, how well your digestion is functioning, and how you're dealing with stress. After your discussion, his pulse examination, and his observation of your physical attributes, your Ayurvedic specialist will make recommendations for you to incorporate into the foundational aspects of your life such as sleeping, eating, and exercising.

Getting a Good Night's Sleep

A good night's sleep is important for your overall health, and you can allow nature's clock to help support your sleep. The hours of 6–10 p.m. naturally have the qualities of kapha. So if you can fall asleep by 10 p.m. the qualities pervasive in the outside world will help you drift into sleep. The hours from 10 p.m.–2 a.m. are characterized as pitta time, so if you aren't asleep before 10 p.m., your body and mind may be influenced by nature's fiery qualities, which will make it harder for you to fall asleep. Because it's pitta time from 10 p.m.–2 a.m., this is the time of night when your body would like to be digesting. If you're sleeping, it's a great time for your body to be able to focus on digesting everything you've taken in during the day while you are resting your senses.

If you have trouble falling asleep, your Ayurvedic specialist can make some recommendations for what to do to help you ease into sleep. One thing she may recommend is self-massage *(see image on page 5 of the insert)*.

BEDTIME SELF-MASSAGE WITH WARM OIL
1. Heat sesame oil for the vata and kapha body types and coconut oil for the pitta types until it's warm to the touch.
2. With slow, soothing strokes, massage your feet with the warm oil.

3. Wash your hands and cover your feet with socks do you don't stain your bedsheets with oil.
4. Massage warm oil along the brow line and at the crown of your head as you take deep, soothing breaths.

Along with self-massage, your specialist may recommend that you try certain herbs, tea, or warm milk before crawling into bed. What she recommends will depend on what she determines is causing you to be imbalanced and unable to fall asleep.

A Good Time to Wake Up

Nature supports your falling asleep and your waking up. Vata time is 2 a.m.–6 a.m., which is the time when people may find themselves naturally waking up even if they'd rather be sleeping. Waking up before 6 a.m. (or sunrise) is ideal because 6 a.m.–10 a.m. is associated with kapha. If you wait until after sunrise to wake up, you'll be struggling to wake up during nature's kapha time. You'll feel the qualities of that time of day, which are sluggish, heavy, and unmotivated as you start your day. If you wake up during vata time, you'll be assisted by those qualities that support the movement of mind and body.

Recommendations for Eating

Your Ayurvedic specialist will recommend whole foods you can gravitate toward and foods that would be better for you to avoid, based on how you are when she sees you. This will change a little bit when the seasons change, and as the doshas in you become balanced and imbalanced based on various factors.

RETHINKING YOUR MAIN MEALTIME

Because 10 a.m.–2 p.m. has pitta qualities, this is the best time to eat your biggest meal. You'll likely be hungry at this time and ready for good digestion because of the fiery qualities of pitta. This fiery time of day supports digestion.

In addition to certain foods, your specialist will likely recommend herbs, teas, oil, powders, and spices for you to add to or eliminate from your diet. All the recommendations are natural and you can stock your kitchen with them so they are easily accessible when you're cooking and eating.

When cooking for an entire family, if you have a family of various constitutions, you can make recipes that are tridoshic—good for balancing all doshas.

Getting Exercise

Movement is very important for your body. It lubricates the joints, aids in digestion, keeps bones strong, helps the flow of fluids in the body, and can be used as an aid for balancing your doshas. Your specialist will take into consideration your constitution, your symptoms, your time of life, and the time of year when she recommends exercise for you. One thing for you to keep in mind is that like increases like and opposites balance. So, for example, if you are predominantly pitta, in your pitta stage of life, and it's summertime, you'll want to avoid vigorous exercise in the heat of the day because that will aggravate pitta in you.

Alternative Therapies

There are alternative therapies that your Ayurvedic specialist may recommend to support your health. Some alternative therapies that support the Ayurvedic lifestyle are Ayurvedic bodywork (massage with warm, herbalized oil), marma balancing therapy (energy work), yoga, meditation, and aromatherapy.

An Ongoing Relationship with Your Specialist/ Practitioner

For continued health and vitality, you can stay in consistent touch with your Ayurvedic specialist. As you experience change in your life, in your mental and physical state, and with age, you can make modifications in your diet and lifestyle. As seasons change, too, you will make some adjustments.

Sustaining Health by Supporting Yourself Daily

When you follow Ayurveda's wisdom as your primary model for healthy living, your focus is on maintaining strong immunity through your diet and lifestyle choices. Instead of waiting until you're sick to focus on taking care of yourself, you maintain your body, mind, and heart so that they can perform their functions to keep you healthy and happy.

For you, this may be a completely new way of thinking about health, and it might seem hard to imagine the real benefit of preventive care. If so, try to imagine that you are preventing illness the same way you prevent your car from breaking down. You get regular oil changes to prevent serious mechanical problems. You fill your car with gas before it becomes empty. You can do the same thing for your health and your body.

In Partnership with Your Practitioner

As you notice changes in your health, or if you have questions, keep in touch with your practitioner. She can continue to make recommendations as you and your life circumstances shift and change. You two will be working together in partnership for your sustained health. To be able to help both you and your practitioner support your health, you can:

- Notice how your body feels, what your mood is like, how your sleep is, how your digestion is, and how your mind is working.
- Follow the recommendations from your practitioner, and be consistent.
- Trust your instincts if something isn't feeling right to you.
- Have positive, healing intentions around your body and heart, mind the food you prepare, and follow the advice of your specialist.
- Envision yourself whole, healed, vital, strong, and radiant.

The relationship between you and your Ayurvedic specialist is an important part of your healing. Make sure you are feeling comfortable with her and that you trust her.

In addition to your specialist's advice and support, your health depends on your commitment to making healthy choices, and your belief in your ability to be well. You really are the one who heals yourself, and your Ayurvedic practitioner guides you and supports you along the way.

Index